SHAHRAD TAHERI
THE HAMMERSMITH HOSPI"

Baillière's
CLINICAL
GASTROENTEROLOGY
INTERNATIONAL PRACTICE AND RESEARCH

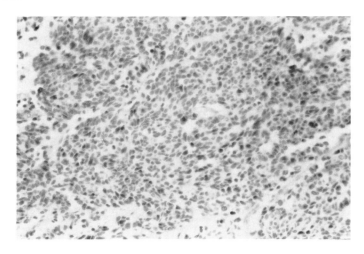

Figure 2. In contrast with Figure 1, this haematoxylin and eosin-stained section of an oseophageal small cell carcinoma shows cells with very little cytoplasm and moderately pleomorphic nuclei.

histological pattern, histology is not a significant aid in assessing tumour prognosis.

Some endocrine tumours of the gut, when well differentiated, have a histological appearance which is sufficiently characteristic to allow identification solely on the basis of conventional histology (e.g. somatostatin-producing duodenal tumours) (Figure 3). For most tumours, however, additional histological screening is necessary.

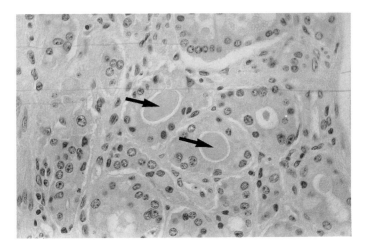

Figure 3. The typical appearance of a somatostatin-rich neuroendocrine tumour of the duodenum is shown in this haematoxylin and eosin-stained section. The main features are the acinar formation of some of the tumour cells and the presence of psammomatous bodies (arrows).

Classification

An early classification of gastrointestinal endocrine tumours separated them into those of the fore-, mid- and hindgut (Williams and Sandler, 1963). This was only of limited help in assessing tumour pathology and was superseded by a system based on histological patterns (Soga and Tazawa, 1971). In this classification, endocrine tumours, at that time referred to solely as 'carcinoids', were assessed as having one or a mixture of the following histological appearances: (A) solid nest or insular; (B) trabecular; (C) glandular; (D) undifferentiated. Later work by a number of endocrine pathologists, most notably Professors Enrico Solcia and Carlo Capella, at the University of Pavia, and Professors Gunter Kloppel and Philipp Heitz, now at Kiel and Zurich, respectively, established classifications based on the histology, site, function and biology of gastrointestinal endocrine tumours and the latest revision was published recently (Capella et al, 1995).

Morphological investigation

Histochemistry

Argyrophilia is a feature of most endocrine cells and is based on the ability of secretory granules to take up and retain silver salts. A chemical is added to reduce the silver, which is precipitated as a black deposit in the cells (Grimelius, 1968) (Figure 4). Some identification of the specific product is possible using stains for argentaffinity, such as the Masson–Fontana technique (Lillie, 1954), as in these silver salts are taken up by granules and, if the amine serotonin (5-hydroxytryptamine) is present, they are reduced. Other histochemical methods which stain endocrine granules,

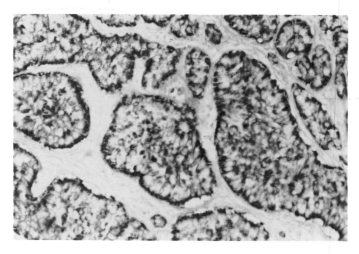

Figure 4. Argyrophilia in a section of an appendiceal carcinoid tumour demonstrated by the silver impregnation technique of Grimelius.

such as the masked metachromasia (Solcia et al, 1968) and lead haematoxylin (Solcia et al, 1969) techniques, are rarely used nowadays.

Conventional electron microscopy

Electron microscopy, which provided crucial information allowing the initial classification of normal endocrine cells and their tumours in the gut (Solcia et al, 1979), remains a valuable tool in the histological investigation of endocrine tumours. Identification of endocrine tumours is usually achieved by immunocytochemistry at the light microscopic level (see below) but ultrastructural analysis can provide crucial information, for example where the levels of stored product are too low to be detected by immunocytochemistry or where only limited tissue is available for investigation, as with a needle biopsy. Examination of the general ultrastructure of the cells can also help in assessing tumour status.

Immunocytochemistry

The major advance in the histological investigation of endocrine tumours occurred with the development of easily reproducible immunocytochemical methods and the wide availability of specific, well-characterized antibodies to markers of endocrine differentiation (see Polak and Van Noorden (1986) for review). Techniques such as the peroxidase anti-peroxidase (PAP) (Sternberger, 1979) and avidin–biotin–peroxidase complex (ABC) (Hsu et al, 1981) methods provide sensitive means to detect endocrine cell products and are widely used in routine laboratories. Immunostaining of endocrine tumours can also be carried out at the ultrastructural level (see Bishop and Polak (1992) for review). Antibodies are available to a number of proteins which are specific to endocrine cells and, thereby, serve as a means to identify tumours as endocrine. These can be divided into cytosolic and granular markers and their details are provided in Table 1. Most commercial

Table 1. General markers of neuroendocrine differentiation.

Peptide or protein	Other names or forms	Cell fraction	Neuroendocrine tumours
Chromogranins	3 forms A, B and C	Secretory granule	All types
Human chorionic gonadotrophin	a and b chains	?	Various
Neural cell adhesion molecule	–	Cell surface	Neural, lung? others
Neuroproteins	–	Neurofilaments	Mainly neural; some other types
Neuron-specific enolase	–	Cytosol	All types
Protein gene product 9.5	–	Cytosol	Mainly neural
7B2	APPG	Secretory granules	Several types
Antigens from small synaptic vesicles			
Synaptobrevin	VAMP-1	Secretory granules	?
Synaptophysin	P38	Secretory granules	All types
P_{65} protein	–	Secretory granules	?

APPG, anterior pituitary peptide of pig.

antibodies available to these proteins are reliable but, as the expression of the proteins can vary with the activity of the tumour or the type of tissue processing used, it is best to stain for at least one cytosolic and one granular marker. An argyrophil stain (e.g. Grimelius'; see above) and, when serotonin production is suspected, an argentaffin stain (e.g. Masson–Fontana's; see above) are useful adjuncts to immunocytochemistry.

Identification of particular gut endocrine tumour types can be achieved by immunostaining of specific products (Table 2). Neoplastic endocrine cells can exhibit altered patterns of peptide synthesis, with production and secretion of abnormal molecular forms. Therefore, when attempting to characterize an endocrine tumour using immunocytochemistry, it is important to use antibodies raised against not only the established, bio-active form of a certain peptide but also other derivatives of its precursor. In addition, there are antibodies available to proliferation markers which can be used in the assessment of tumour prognosis. One of the most popular is the monoclonal antibody MIB-1 which recognizes the cell-cycle-associated protein Ki-67 (Brown and Gatter, 1990). Varied results have been obtained with this antibody which was useful in distinguishing between parathyroid adenomas and carcinomas (Lloyd et al, 1995) but showed a high degree of overlap in proliferative index between benign and malignant tumours of the gastroenteropancreatic tract (von Herbay et al, 1991).

Table 2. Main neuroendocrine tumours of the gastrointestinal tract.

Site	Major cell type	Product(s)
Oesophagus	EC	Serotonin (rare)
	P	?ACTH, calcitonin
Fundus	EC	Serotonin (rare)
	ECL	?Histamine
	D_1–P	?
	Inappropriate	ACTH
Antrum	G	Gastrin
	D	Somatostatin (rare)
	P–D_1	?
	Inappropriate	ACTH
Small intestine	C–IG	Gastrin
	D	Somatostatin
	?Paraganglia	Somatostatin, PP
	EC	Serotonin, tachykinins
	P	?
Large intestinal	L	Glucagon and related peptides, PYY
	EC	Serotonin (rare)
	D	Somatostatin (rare)

ACTH, adrenocorticotrophic hormone; PP, pancreatic polypeptide; PYY, peptide tyrosine tyrosine.

In situ hybridization

Hybridization of complementary nucleotide sequences, for so long the province of molecular biologists, has been adapted for use on tissue preparations and is being applied increasingly in the investigation and routine diagnosis of endocrine tumours. Labelled complementary nucleic acid sequences are applied to tissues where, under optimized conditions, they form stable hybrids with endogenous DNA or RNA (see Polak and McGee (1990) for review). Isotopic labelling of sequences provides a sensitive means of localizing endogenous nucleotides but gives poor resolution and obvious safety hazards. Non-isotopic labels are proving more popular and include biotin (Langer et al, 1981) and digoxigenin (Herrington et al, 1990) (Figure 5). In situ hybridization allows identification of poorly granulated tumours and can provide information on the functional activity of the cells.

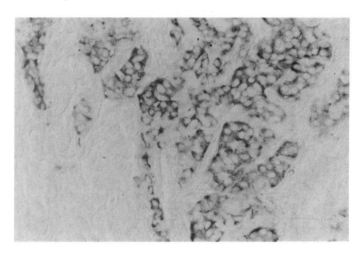

Figure 5. The presence and distribution of insulin mRNA in a section of a pancreatic B cell tumour shown by in situ hybridization using digoxigenin-labelled insulin cRNA.

GASTROINTESTINAL ENDOCRINE TUMOURS

Oesophagus

Endocrine tumours are rarely found in the oesophagus and mainly comprise neuroendocrine or small cell carcinomas (Reyes et al, 1980; Briggs and Ibrahim, 1983). These tumours, which have also been described in stomach (Solcia et al, 1986) and colon (Chejfec and Gould, 1977), arise from proto-endocrine cells and are not associated with any clinical syndrome. Typically, histology shows sheets of small cells with round or spindle-shaped nuclei and scant cytoplasm. Areas of necrosis are common. Small cell carcinomas are poorly granulated and, with the exception of neuron-specific enolase, usually show little immunoreactivity for endocrine cell products.

Stomach

Most gastric endocrine tumours arise in the oxyntic mucosa and, although their histology has been studied extensively, their functions have yet to be characterized fully. In conditions of hypo- or achlorhydria and hyper-gastrinaemia, for example in association with chronic atrophic gastritis, there can be hyperplasia of endocrine cells and formation of extra-epithelial clusters, so-called microcarcinoids (Figure 6). These growths are composed mostly of enterochromaffin-like (ECL) cells (see Polak and Bloom (1988) for review). Against a background of hypergastrinaemia, well-differentiated microcarcinoids, less than 1 cm in diameter, tend to be benign. However, a series of similarly well-differentiated growths, presenting without hypergastrinaemia, was found to show metastases in more than 60% of cases (Rindi et al, 1993). In order to allow some prediction of the behaviour of these lesions, a detailed classification has been produced of the various steps in the pathogenesis of malignant endocrine tumours of the non-antral stomach, from simple hyperplasia to invasive tumour (Solcia et al, 1988).

Histologically, ECL cell tumours usually have a nested or trabecular architecture. No peptide has been identified in normal or neoplastic ECL cells but they are known to produce histamine in rodents and there have been isolated reports of the presence of histamine in normal human ECL cells (Lonroth et al, 1990) and of raised levels being detected in the circulation of patients with ECL cell tumours (Sandler and Snow, 1958).

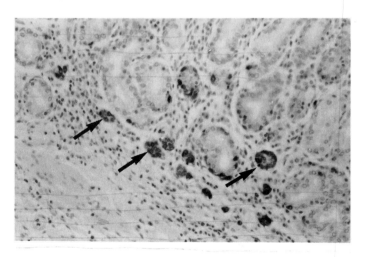

Figure 6. Immunocytochemistry for chromogranin, a general marker of neuroendocrine differentiation, shows the presence of extra-epithelial clusters of enterochromaffin-like cells (arrows) in inflamed gastric mucosa.

These tumours typically display strong immunoreactivity for chromogranin and neuron-specific enolase and are argyrophils.

The gastric antrum–pylorus is the major site for gastrin (G) cells but very few gastric G cell tumours have been described. Most gastrin-producing tumours are found in the upper small intestine (see later) or pancreas. When they do present in the stomach, these tumours are usually associated with the typical Zollinger–Ellison syndrome (ZES) or gastrinoma syndrome.

Small intestine

G cell tumours are the most common endocrine tumour of the upper small intestine and the ZES is the only clinical syndrome due to hypersecretion from endocrine tumours in this region of the gut (Figure 7). Around 60% of patients with multiple endocrine neoplasia type 1 (MEN 1) have full-blown ZES or raised levels of circulating gastrin (Thompson et al, 1989; Kloppel et al, 1986). For a long time, it was thought that this hypergastrinaemia was the result of a pancreatic G cell tumour; a feature of MEN 1 is widespread pathology of the endocrine pancreas with nesidioblastosis and multiple microscopic adenomata, in addition to larger tumours which can be detected by scanning techniques. Partial pancreatectomy often failed to lower serum gastrin levels (Deveney et al, 1983; Malagelada et al, 1983) and immunocytochemical analysis of resected pancreatic lesions usually provides no evidence for gastrin production (Kloppel et al, 1986; Bordi et al, 1987; Pilato et al, 1988; Pipeleers-Marichal et al, 1990). It appears, therefore, that G cell tumours, associated with MEN 1 or sporadic (Delcore et al, 1988; Thompson et al, 1989), are most frequent in the duodenum.

Non-functioning G cell tumours are mainly benign and those associated with the ZES show low to moderate malignant potential; in a series of 103

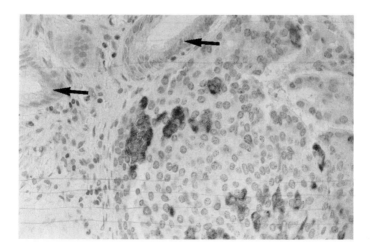

Figure 7. Gastrin immunoreactivity in a malignant neuroendocrine tumour infiltrating the duodenal mucosa (arrows show mucosal epithelium).

duodenal G cell tumours associated with ZES, 38% were reported to be malignant (Hoffmann et al, 1973).

Tumours composed almost exclusively of D (somatostatin) cells (Figure 8) and mainly present in the peri-ampullary region are a comparatively recently recognized entity (Dayal et al, 1983; Griffiths et al, 1984). They appear in the literature under a variety of terms, including psammomatous somatostatinoma and somatostatin-rich glandular carcinoid. These tumours are not associated with any of the symptoms sometimes attributed to pancreatic D cell tumours, such as steatorrhoea, diarrhoea and diabetes mellitus, and they usually present as the cause of obstructive biliary disease. In general, the tumours are composed of regular cells arranged in glands or acini with psammoma bodies in the lumina. This glandular structure can lead to misdiagnosis of these tumours as adenocarcinomas. In contrast with other endocrine tumours of the upper small intestine, D cell tumours show a moderate to high rate of malignancy.

They can present in association with phaeochromocytoma and von Recklinghausen's disease in the MEN 2 syndrome (Dayal et al, 1986; Stamm et al, 1986).

Gangliocytic paragangliomas are rare neuroendocrine lesions of the duodenum and are benign tumours composed of fully differentiated ganglion cells, epithelial endocrine cells and Schwann-like spindle cells. Somatostatin has been detected in both neural and endocrine cell types using immunocytochemistry and pancreatic polypeptide was found in the endocrine cells (Hamid et al, 1986). The exact histogenesis of gangliocytic paragangliomas is unknown. A possible relationship between the epithelial, glandular D cell tumour (described above) and this paraganglioma has been suggested, with the former representing a purely epithelial form of the latter

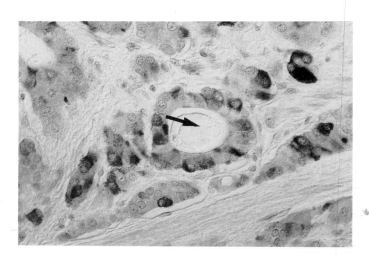

Figure 8. Section of a peri-ampullary neuroendocrine tumour showing immunoreactivity for somato-statin. A psammomatous body can be seen (arrow).

Sandler M & Snow PJD (1958) An atypical carcinoid tumour secreting 5-hydroxytryptophan. *Lancet* **i:** 137–139.

Soga J & Tazawa K (1971) Pathologic analysis of carcinoids. Histologic re-evaluation of 62 cases. *Cancer* **28:** 990–998.

Solcia E, Vassallo G & Capella C (1968) Selective staining of endocrine cells by basic dyes after acid hydrolysis. *Stain Technology* **43:** 257–263.

Solcia E, Capella C & Vassallo G (1969) Lead haematoxylin as a stain for endocrine cells: significance of staining and comparison with other selective methods. *Histochemie* **20:** 116–126.

Solcia E, Capella C, Buffa R et al (1979) Endocrine cells of the gastrointestinal tract and related tumours. *Pathobiology Annual* **9:** 163–203.

Solcia E, Capella C, Sessa F et al (1986) Gastric carcinoids and related endocrine growths. *Digestion* **35:** 3–22.

Solcia E, Bordi C, Creutzfeldt W et al (1988) Classification of non-antral gastric endocrine growths in man. *Digestion* **41:** 185–200.

Solcia E, Rindi G, Sessa F et al (1993) Endocrine tumours of the gastrointestinal tract. In Polak JM (ed.) *Diagnostic Histopathology of Neuroendocrine Tumours*, pp123–149. Edinburgh: Churchill Livingstone.

Stamm B, Hedinger E & Saremaslami P (1986) Duodenal and ampullary carcinoid tumours. A report of 12 cases with pathobiological characteristics, polypeptide content and relation to the MEN1 syndrome and von Recklinghausen's disease (neurofibromatosis). *Virchows Archiv A, Pathological Anatomy and Histopathology* **408:** 475–489.

Stephens M, Williams GT, Jasani B & Williams ED (1987) Synchronous duodenal neuroendocrine tumours in von Recklinghausen's disease—case report of co-existing gangliocytic paraganglioma and somatostatin-rich glandular carcinoid. *Histopathology* **11:** 1331–1340.

Sternberger LA (1979) The unlabelled antibody peroxidase anti-peroxidase (PAP) method. In Sternberger LA (ed.) *Immunocytochemistry*, pp104–169. New York: John Wiley.

Thompson NW, Vinik AI & Eckhauser FE (1989) Microgastrinomas of the duodenum: a cause of failed operations of the Zollinger–Ellison syndrome. *Annuals of Surgery* **121:** 195–205.

Thompson EA, Fleming KA, Evans DJ et al (1990) Gastric endocrine cells share a clonal origin with other gut cell lineages. *Development* **110:** 477–481.

Williams ED & Sandler M (1963) The classification of carcinoid tumours. *Lancet* **i:** 238–239.

2

Peptide receptors in gut endocrine tumours

WOUTER W. DE HERDER
LEO J. HOFLAND
AART-JAN VAN DER LELY
STEVEN W. J. LAMBERTS

Pancreatic islet cell tumours and carcinoids may produce one or more peptide hormones. These tumoral products are released into the circulation and subsequently transported to various target organs on which they exert their action. Generally, this excessive hormone production will be reflected by a characteristic clinical syndrome. It is possible to measure the levels of most peptides in the blood, providing suitable markers for disease stage and endocrinological activity (Reubi, 1993). In addition, the high expression of receptors for some peptides by these tumours provides other valuable tumour markers. One of these peptides is somatostatin and the research field into this peptide hormone and its structurally related analogues has rapidly expanded over the last decade (Reubi, 1993).

SOMATOSTATIN, ITS RECEPTORS AND ITS EFFECTS

Somatostatin, originally termed somatotrophin release inhibitory factor (SRIF), is a small cyclic peptide hormone, which is present in humans in the molecular forms SRIF-14 (consisting of 14 amino acids) and SRIF-28 (28 amino acids) (Figure 1) (Brazeau et al, 1973; Pradayrol et al, 1980). SRIF has diverse biological effects in different organ systems. In the exocrine and endocrine pancreas, locally synthesized SRIF may exert an endocrine or paracrine effect. These effects are mediated through specific SRIF receptors (ssts) on the target tissues. The presence of ssts has also been demonstrated throughout the human gastrointestinal mucosa. The gastrointestinal transit time, secretion of intestinal hormones by intestinal endocrine cells, the peptide-induced secretion of intestinal fluid and the resorption of intestinal fluid can be inhibited through the action of SRIF on these receptors (Lamberts et al, 1996).

Ssts are membrane-associated receptors consisting of a single polypeptide chain with seven transmembrane domains: extracellular domains with ligand binding sites and intracellular domains with sites linked to the

Baillière's Clinical Gastroenterology—
Vol. 10, No. 4, December 1996
ISBN 0-7020-2186-5
0950-3528/96/040571 + 17 $12.00/00

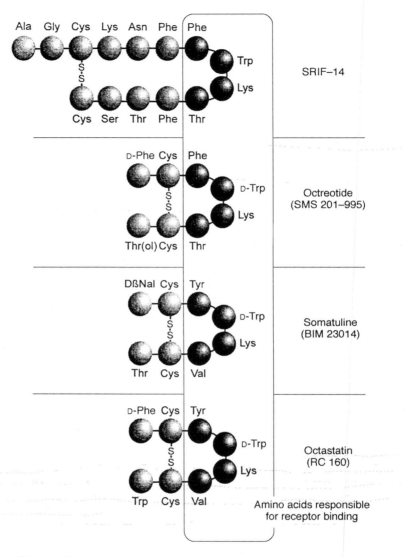

Figure 1. Comparative amino acid sequence of somatostatin and its analogues.

activation of second messengers. They belong to the family of G-protein-coupled receptors (Reisine and Bell, 1995). A large variety of primary tumours and their metastases can also express a high density of ssts (Lamberts, 1988; Lamberts et al, 1991). Recently, five different sst subtypes have been cloned and characterized. These receptor subtypes have been named sst$_{1-5}$ (Hoyer et al, 1995). In humans, the genes encoding for the sst subtypes have a distinct chromosomal localization and their mRNAs have a tissue-specific expression pattern. Additionally, it has been shown that few, if any, tumours express only a single sst subtype mRNA, while most express multiple sst subtype mRNAs. However, sst_2 mRNA predominance is found in most tumours (see below). Although the different sst subtypes are 40–60% structurally homologous, each sst subtype potentially mediates different biological actions of SRIF (Reubi, 1995a).

SOMATOSTATIN, ITS OCTAPEPTIDE ANALOGUES AND THEIR RECEPTORS

For therapeutic purposes, SRIF needs to be administered by the intravenous (i.v.) route owing to its short half-life (less than 3 min). The peptide has simultaneous effects in different organ systems, which sometimes offers more a disadvantage, rather than an advantage. Furthermore, post-infusion rebound hypersecretion of hormones does occur. Therefore, structural analogues of SRIF that do not have these drawbacks have been synthesized via step-by-step modification of SRIF. These analogues are relatively resistant to proteolytic enzymes, which has resulted in longer half-lives. Octreotide (SMS 201-995, Sandostatin) (Figure 1) is a synthetic octapeptide, which retains the sequence residues 7–10 of SRIF-14 (Phe–Trp–Lys–Thr, essential for receptor binding) and has incorporated the Trp residue in the D configuration. Octreotide has a half-life in the circulation of about 113 min. The drug can be administered by multiple subcutaneous (s.c.) injections, or by continuous s.c. infusion, and by the i.v. route, either as a single injection or as a continuous infusion over many hours or days. A slow-release depot intramuscular (i.m.) formulation of octreotide (Sandostatin-LAR) is expected to be available for clinical use in the near future. This drug has to be administered once every 4 weeks (Lamberts et al, 1996). Somatuline (BIM 23014) (Figure 1) is another synthetic and also cyclic octapeptide with a similar therapeutic profile to octreotide. It can be given by the same routes of administration as octreotide. A slow-release i.m. depot formulation (Lanreotide, BIM-LA), which needs to be administered every 10–15 days, is currently available. RC 160 (Octastatin, Vapreotide) (Figure 1) is a synthetic octapeptide, which is at present undergoing pharmacological testing. Both BIM 23014 and RC 160 are Tyr^3/Val^6-substituted SRIF analogues, which also have substitutions at positions 1 (DβNal for DPhe) and 8 (Trp for Thr(ol)) respectively of the molecule (Figure 1). Interestingly, the five cloned sst subtypes show a distinct pharmacological binding profile for these SRIF analogues in comparison with that of native SRIF. Both SRIF-14 and SRIF-28 bind with high affinities to all sst subtypes. Octreotide, BIM 23014 and RC 160 have comparable binding profiles and bind with a high affinity to sst_2 and sst_5, show a low affinity to sst_3, and no affinity to sst_1 and sst_4. Although slight differences have been reported in the action on tumour cell growth (Liebow et al, 1989) and in the affinity for SRIF-14 binding sites (Srkalovic et al, 1990) as well as in the potency (Hofland et al, 1994) of these octapeptide analogues, no major differences can be expected between their therapeutic effects.

CLINICAL RELEVANCE OF SOMATOSTATIN RECEPTOR EXPRESSION IN CARCINOIDS AND PANCREATIC ENDOCRINE TUMOURS

Apart from the usefulness as a tumour marker, the expression of ssts by human tumours has other important clinical implications, such as

- inhibition of tumoral peptide hormone secretion by somatostatin (analogues) and
- inhibition of tumoral growth by somatostatin (analogues).

In peptide-hormone-secreting carcinoids and islet cell tumours, ssts mediate the inhibition of hormone secretion by SRIF (analogues). In up to 70% of these patients, clinical symptomatology can be controlled by the chronic administration of one of the octapeptide analogues (Lamberts et al, 1996). A highly significant correlation has been demonstrated between the sst status and the inhibition of hormonal secretion by these tumours by octreotide in vivo, as well as their effects on tumour cell growth in culture (for an example see Figure 2 (A–E) (Reubi, 1995a). In sst-negative tumours, octreotide had no effect on the hormonal production (Lamberts et al, 1990; Reubi et al, 1990). The inhibitory effects of SRIF (analogues), mediated via ssts, are linked with several intracellular effector systems. Most pronounced are the effects on adenylyl cyclase, resulting in a decrease in the intracellular cAMP levels, but SRIF also reduces Ca^{2+} influxes, resulting in reduced intracellular Ca^{2+} levels, while SRIF stimulates tyrosine phosphatase activity in a number of tissues (Hofland and Lamberts, 1996). In conclusion, the expression of ssts by islet cell tumours and carcinoids is essential for the control of hormonal hypersecretion by the octapeptide analogues. However, within months of continuous administration, insensitivity to octreotide develops in almost all patients. This is probably due to a preferential outgrowth of sst-negative tumour cell clones, although down-regulation of ssts might also play a role (Lamberts et al, 1988).

SRIF (analogues) exert(s) an antiproliferative action on sst-positive tumours. Several mechanisms of action might play a role in this effect (Reubi and Laissue, 1995):

1. through inhibition of the secretion of tumour-growth-promoting hormones (growth hormone (GH), insulin, gastrointestinal hormones) in an endocrine fashion;
2a. through direct or indirect (via GH) inhibition of the production and biological activity of insulin-like growth factor I (IGF-I);
 b. through regulation of the IGF-binding proteins (IGF-BPs);
 c. through other tumour growth factors;
3. through effects on angiogenesis and tumour blood supply (Reubi et al, 1994a);

(A)

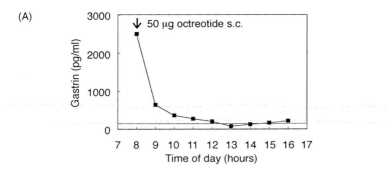

(B)

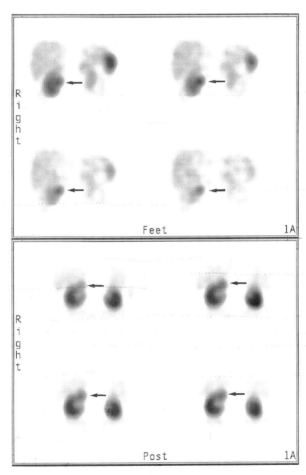

Figure 2. A forty-year-old woman with diarrhoea, hyperacidity and recurrent multiple duodenal peptic ulcers, which were refractory to therapy with H_2 receptor antagonists on the basis of the Zollinger–Ellison syndrome. (A) Effect of a single subcutaneous injection of 50 µg octreotide on serum gastrin levels in vivo. Octreotide successfully suppressed the pathologically elevated gastrin levels to values within, or close to the normal range (Normal: gastrin < 150 pg/ml). (B) Coronal (top panel) and transverse (bottom panel) single photon emission computer tomography at 24 hours after intravenous injection of ^{111}In-labelled pentetreotide showing a lesion with increased uptake of radioactivity located ventromedially from the right kidney (arrows). (Courtesy of Dr H.Y. Oei and Professor Dr E.P. Krenning).

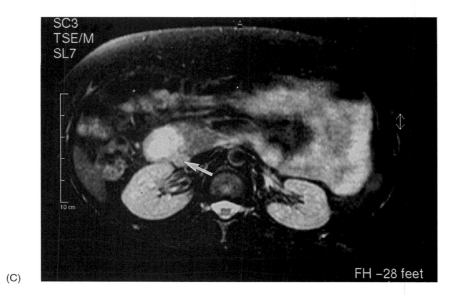

(C)

(D)

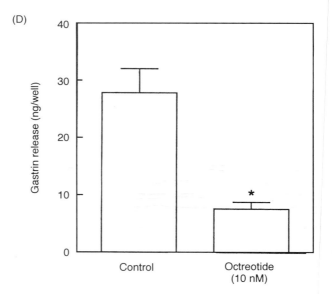

Figure 2. (C) Abdominal magnetic resonance imaging: T1-weighted images in the transverse plane showing the primary gastrinoma (diameter 0.5 cm in the transverse plane) located in the pancreatic head, situated medially and dorsally to the duodenum and in the close proximity of the right kidney (arrows). (Courtesy of Dr J. Stoker.) At operation, a 0.5 cm × 1.5 cm gastrinoma was enucleated from the pancreatic head. (D) Effects of octreotide on gastrinoma cells in culture. Cells were dissociated and cultured in minimal essential medium with 10% fetal calf serum as described previously (Hofland et al, 1994). 50 000 cells were seeded per well (24-well plate) and cultured for 3 days in the above medium. Thereafter, the medium was changed and a 3-day incubation without or with octreotide (10 nM) was performed in quadruplicate. After 3 days the medium was collected and stored at −20 °C until determination of gastrin concentrations by radioimmunoassay as described (Hofland et al, 1994). Values are the mean ±SE of four wells. *$P < 0.01$ versus control cells without octreotide.

(E)

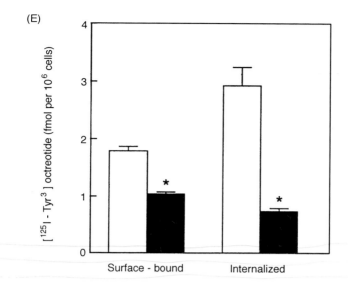

(F)

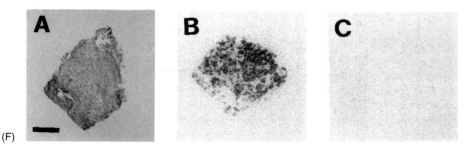

Figure 2. (E) Internalization of octreotide into gastrinoma cells. Cells were dissociated and cultured in minimal essential medium with 10% fetal calf serum as described previously (Hofland et al, 1994). 10^6 cells were seeded per well (six-well plate) and cultured for 3 days in the above medium. After 3 days the medium was changed and the cells were incubated for 4 hours with [^{125}I-Tyr^3]octreotide (0.1 nM) without (open bars) or with (filled bars) excess (1 μM) unlabelled octreotide. Thereafter, the amount of surface-bound and internalized radioactivity was determined by the acid-washing method, as described previously (Hofland et al, 1995a). Values are the mean ±SE of four wells. *$P < 0.01$ versus control cells without unlabelled octreotide. (F) Somatostatin receptors in the gastrinoma tissue. A: hematoxylin–eosin stained section; bar, 1mm. B: autoradiogram showing total binding of ^{125}I-labelled Tyr^3-octreotide. Note the labelling of the tumour cells with the radioligand. C: autoradiogram showing non-specific binding (in presence of 1 μM unlabelled octreotide).

4. through direct anti-proliferative effects on the tumour by binding to specific sst subtypes, resulting in stimulation of a tyrosine phosphatase and reversion of the growth-promoting activity of the tyrosine-kinase-linked group of oncogenes (mediated via sst_2), or reduction of Ca^{2+} influxes (mediated via sst_5) (Buscail et al, 1995);
5. through cell-cycle-dependent induction of apoptosis (Srikant, 1995);
6. through the inhibition of local paracrine- and/or autocrine-secreted growth factors.

Octreotide significantly inhibited the growth of an sst-positive human carcinoid (BON) xenotransplanted into a nude mouse (Evers et al, 1991). However, octreotide stimulated growth of these BON cells in a dose-dependent fashion in vitro (Ishizuka et al, 1992). Therefore, an as-yet unexplained direct growth-stimulatory effect might be responsible for the negative therapeutic effects of octreotide on tumour growth observed in some carcinoids.

Octreotide therapy in patients with metastatic carcinoids resulted in objective tumour regression in less than 20% and temporary stabilization of tumour growth in the majority of patients. In some patients, radiographic evidence of increased intratumoral necrosis was found (Lamberts et al, 1991, 1996). In conclusion, octapeptide analogues may control tumour growth of part of the sst-positive islet cell tumours and carcinoids.

IN VITRO AND IN VIVO DEMONSTRATION OF SOMATOSTATIN RECEPTOR EXPRESSION IN CARCINOIDS AND PANCREATIC ENDOCRINE TUMOURS

Ssts have been demonstrated in vitro by radioligand binding assays in tissue homogenates, or by quantitative receptor autoradiography of tissue sections, using [^{125}I-Tyr^3]octreotide, [^{125}I-Tyr^{11}]SRIF-14, or [^{125}I-LTT]SRIF-28 (for an example see Figure 2(E)) (Reubi et al, 1994b; Reubi, 1995a). Reubi and coworkers have found that the majority of well-differentiated carcinoids express ssts, whereas ssts are often absent on less-differentiated, more aggressively growing 'atypical carcinoids'. This may be put into relation with the observation that in some other neoplastic tissues (except for meningiomas and renal cell carcinomas) an inverse relation was found between the presence of ssts and receptors for epidermal growth factor, which is an important mitogen (Reubi et al, 1992a; Ahlman et al, 1993).

Sst subtype mRNA expression in human tissues has been studied in vitro using in situ hybridization, Northern blotting, ribonuclease protection assays and by amplification by reverse transcription and the polymerase chain reaction (RT–PCR) (Reubi, 1995a). Reubi and coworkers have studied sst_1, sst_2 and sst_3 mRNA expression in carcinoids and islet cell tumours by in situ hybridization. These results were compared with those obtained by quantitative receptor autoradiography with [^{125}I-Tyr^3]octreotide and [^{125}I-LTT]SRIF-28 on adjacent sections of the tumours. Expression of mRNA for sst_1 was found in five of 11 carcinoids and in three of five islet cell tumours. The mRNA for sst_2 was expressed in seven of 11 carcinoids and in three of five islet cell tumours and mRNA for sst_3 was only expressed in two of 11 carcinoids and in four of five islet cell tumours. Autoradiography of carcinoids and islet cell tumours expressing mRNA for sst_2 showed strong positivity of the tumours for [^{125}I-Tyr^3]octreotide. However, in one carcinoid, only expression of mRNA for sst_1 was found, but not for sst_2 and sst_3. Autoradiography of this tumour was strongly positive for [^{125}I-LTT]SRIF-28, but negative for [^{125}I-Tyr^3]octreotide. Therefore, [^{125}I-Tyr^3]octreotide in binding experiments may select among sst_1 and sst_2 those tumours expressing sst_2. One islet cell tumour expressed mRNA for sst_1 and sst_3. Autoradiography of this tumour showed strong positivity for [^{125}I-LTT]SRIF-28, but also for [^{125}I-Tyr^3]octreotide, thereby demonstrating that octreotide also has affinity to sst_3 (Reubi et al, 1994c). Using RT–PCR, Kubota and coworkers studied sst mRNA expression in a glucagonoma, a metastatic glucagonoma, four insulinomas and a carcinoid. The glucagonomas expressed all sst subtype mRNAs except that for sst_5. This was reflected by the fact that in one of these patients treatment with octreotide resulted in a significant decrease of plasma glucagon levels. Sst_1 and sst_4 mRNAs were detected in all four insulinomas, but sst_2 mRNA was detected in three of four tumours and sst_3 mRNA was only detected in two of four tumours. In one carcinoid, sst_1 and sst_4 mRNAs were detected, but not the sst_2, sst_3, and sst_5 mRNAs. In this patient, treatment with octreotide failed to reduce the plasma (sic) 5-hydroxyindole acetic acid levels (Kubota et al, 1994). Using the same molecular biological technique, Vikić–Topic and coworkers have demonstrated the presence of sst_1 and sst_2 mRNAs in 12 of 15 and 14 of 15 carcinoids, respectively, whereas sst_3 and sst_4 mRNAs were only present in two of 15 and one of 15 carcinoids, respectively (Vikić–Topic et al, 1995). In conclusion, there is a heterogeneous expression of the human sst subtype mRNAs in islet cell tumours and carcinoids. In general, there is predominant expression of sst_1 and sst_2 mRNA and little to variable expression of sst_3 and sst_4. The efficacy of the octapeptide analogues seems to be determined by the expression of sst_2 on these tumours.

Tumours and metastases which bear receptors for octapeptide analogues can be visualized in vivo using γ camera pictures obtained after injection of [^{123}I-Tyr^3]octreotide, or [^{111}In]pentetreotide (OctreoScan, Mallinckrodt, Petten, The Netherlands) (Lamberts et al, 1991; Reubi et al, 1992b; Krenning et al, 1993; Kwekkeboom et al, 1993b; Lamberts et al, 1993). In a large European multicentre trial, a total of 350 patients with islet cell tumours and carcinoids has been studied by means of this technique. [^{111}In]pentetreotide scintigraphy was positive in 87% of carcinoids ($N = 184$), 73% of gastrinomas and non-secreting islet cell tumours ($N = 49$, $N = 49$, respectively), 46% of insulinomas ($N = 24$), 88% of VIP-omas ($N = 8$), all five glucagonomas and none of two somatostatinomas (for an example see Figure 2(B) and (C)) (Krenning et al, 1994b; Jamar et al, 1995). In somatostatinomas, the chronic exposure of the tumour to excess endogenous somatostatin may result in down-regulation of ssts

(Krenning et al, 1995). Janson and coworkers studied 30 patients with carcinoids, using [¹¹¹In]pentetreotide scintigraphy (Janson et al, 1994). In 27 patients, accumulation of the radiolabel in tumour deposits was observed. Of these, 22 patients (81%) showed a significant biochemical response to somatostatin analogue treatment, defined as a more than 50% decrease in tumour markers. All patients responding to octreotide therapy were sst scintigraphy positive. Five patients with a positive [¹¹¹In]pentetreotide scintigraphy failed to respond to octapeptide analogues. This might be explained by the high cut-off limit for decrease in tumour markers which was used by these authors. Defining a positive response as a more than 25% decrease in tumour markers limits this series to only two 'non-responding' patients. It has been suggested that these cases may relate to a putative post-sst defect, or to heterogeneous sst_2 and sst_5 distribution on the tumours. None of the three scan-negative patients showed a biochemical response to octapeptide analogue treatment. The tumours in these patients showed a more malignant course of disease. These observations parallel the earlier in vitro findings by Reubi et al (1990), showing that the presence of ssts on these tumours can be used as a marker of differentiation. Sst-negative tumours might constitute a poorly differentiated subgroup of carcinoids, and chemotherapy should be considered in these patients (see below). In conclusion, (1) the in vivo hormonal studies obtained after the administration of SRIF (analogues), (2) the in vitro studies with cultured tumour cells after the administration of SRIF (analogues) and (3) the results of in vivo sst scintigraphy are closely correlated in patients with carcinoids and islet cell tumours. This suggests that a positive scintigram in a patient with an islet cell tumour or carcinoid predicts a therapeutic effect of octapeptide analogues on hormonal hypersecretion by these tumours. Sst scintigraphy, however, is not specific for carcinoids or islet cell tumours, as ssts have also been recognized in vitro and demonstrated in vivo on a variety of other neoplastic tissues, such as other amine precursor uptake and decarboxylation carcinomas, pancreatic and colorectal adenocarcinomas, and lymphomas, but also on non-neoplastic processes, such as granulomas, lesions in autoimmune diseases with systemic involvement, and veins and venules in inflammatory bowel disease (van Hagen et al, 1994; Reubi et al, 1994b; Virgolini et al, 1994). Ssts have also been demonstrated on the peritumoral vasculature system of a number of tumour types. The presence of these vascular ssts seems to be independent of the sst status of the tumour itself (Reubi et al, 1994a; Reubi and Laissue, 1995).

In conclusion, sst scintigraphy is a useful tool in the diagnostic work-up of patients with known islet cell tumours and carcinoids, to localize the primary tumour as well as its metastatic spread. However, in vivo scintigraphy is not suitable for the differential diagnosis of these tumours. With this technique, false negative findings can be produced by

- tumours with low sst density and
- tumours with high endogenous SRIF production.

On the other hand, false positive results can be produced by

- identification of non-neoplastic, sst-positive tissues,
- binding to antibodies against chronically injected octreotide (Kwekkeboom et al, 1993a) and
- binding to ssts on the peritumoral vascular system and lymphocytes.

SOMATOSTATIN-RECEPTOR-MEDIATED INTERNALIZATION OF SOMATOSTATIN (ANALOGUES)

Once activated by binding with octreotide, ssts can be internalized as a receptor–ligand complex into cultured human carcinoid cells (for an example in gastrinoma cells see Figure 2(E)) (Hofland et al, 1995b). In the tumour cell, this complex will be either degraded by lysosomes, or recycled and re-integrated into the cell membrane. Internalization of octreotide may explain the long residence time of radioactivity in sst-positive tumours in vivo in sst scintigraphy. This is of particular importance when radiotherapy of sst-positive metastatic carcinoids and islet cell tumours with α- or β-emitting isotopes coupled to somatostatin (analogues) is considered. The process of internalization might bring the radioligand closer to its target: the nucleus and its DNA. It is at present unclear whether sst_2, sst_5, or both receptor subtypes are involved in this process. Radiotherapy requires a high target-to-background uptake of radioactivity, as the large number of non-neoplastic tissues expressing ssts should not be placed at risk from the cyto-toxic effect of the radioligand. The rapid decrease in blood radioactivity and the predominantly renal clearance of [^{111}In]pentetreotide are advantageous in this respect. However, renal accumulation and the relatively long renal half-life may limit the cumulatively applicable dose of this radioligand. Therapies which potentially lower renal exposure to radiation are currently under investigation (Krenning et al, 1995). The feasibility of this treatment modality might also be improved by up-regulation of targeted ssts. Hofland and coworkers have shown that internalization of [^{125}I-Tyr^3]octreotide into cultured pituitary adenoma cells increased in the presence of low concen-trations of unlabelled octreotide (Hofland et al, 1995a).

Radiotherapy of an sst-positive metastatic glucagonoma, using Auger and conversion electrons emitted by [^{111}In]pentetreotide, has resulted in a transient biochemical response and a transient reduction in the volume of some of the sst-positive metastases (Krenning et al, 1994a).

SOMATOSTATIN RECEPTOR STATUS OF ISLET CELL TUMOURS AND CARCINOIDS: POTENTIAL BENEFITS FOR PATIENT MANAGEMENT

Neuroendocrine malignancies can be treated by surgery with palliative or curative intent. Currently, the following modalities are used: medical therapy with octreotide or interferons, hepatic artery embolization, surgical ligation of the arterial blood supply to the liver, systemic or liver-targeted (single-agent or combination) chemotherapy, external or internal radiotherapy (with radioisotope-coupled somatostatin (analogues)) and combinations of these procedures (Oberg, 1993; Moertel et al, 1994; Oberg et al, 1994). For the selection of the optimal treatment protocol for the individual patient, one has to take into account

1. the general clinical condition of the patient,
2. the course of the disease,
3. the severity of the clinical syndrome related to hormonal hyper-secretion and
4. the tumour burden in combination with
   a. the localization of the primary tumour(s) and
   b. the localization of the metastases.

Knowledge of the sst status of the tumour can be used to optimize the choice of therapy for the individual patient. In some cases, whole-body scintigraphy with [^{111}In]pentetreotide identified more tumour deposits than were found with conventional radiological investigations (Kwekkeboom et al, 1993b; Krenning et al, 1995). This often had a negative impact on tumour staging and resulted in modification of the (pre-operative and/or post-operative) therapeutic approach (Kwekkeboom et al, 1993b; Lebtahi et al, 1994). Patients with tumours limited to the pancreas, or localized in one part of the gastrointestinal tract, or patients with only limited (local) metastatic spread can be potentially cured by surgery alone. In selected cases, resection of solitary liver metastases or partial hepatectomy is feasible (McEntee et al, 1990). [^{111}In]pentetreotide scintigraphy might be used in the follow-up of curatively operated patients, to detect regrowth of tumour remnants or newly occurring metastases at an early stage. However, as already mentioned, this technique has a very high sensitivity for sst-positive tumours, but a low specificity. Importantly, in rare cases, tumours express-ing sst_2 mRNA and binding radiolabelled octreotide and tumours that do not express sst_2, sst_3, and sst_5 and do not bind radiolabelled octreotide may co-exist in one and the same patient (Reubi et al, 1994c, patient 7/TA). In this case, [^{111}In]pentetreotide scintigraphy gives false-negative results.

As already mentioned, treatment with octapeptide analogues improves the quality of life (by alleviating signs and symptoms related to hormonal excess), delays disease progression and improves survival, especially in those patients which cannot be treated by curative surgery alone, or in whom palliative surgery (tumour debulking) has already been performed. [^{111}In]pentetreotide scintigraphy can be used to select patients who are likely to respond to therapy with octapeptide analogues. Negative sst imaging should alert the physician to the presence of a poorly differentiated tumour. In such cases, a tumour biopsy should be taken for histological confirmation. The inconvenience and expense of octreotide therapy should be spared in those patients. Anaplastic tumours show a more aggressive clinical behaviour, but a higher response rate to combination chemotherapy (>65%) than the relatively low response (10%) of well-differentiated tumours (Moertel et al, 1991, 1992).

Radiolabelled octapeptide analogues can also be used in combination with a hand-held radionuclide probe, assisting the surgeon as an intra-abdominal scanning device in the intra-operative search for tumour deposits and allowing for complete removal (Schirmer et al, 1993).

Finally, in cases resistant to all the 'conventional' therapies, (experimental) radiotherapy with radiolabelled chelated somatostatin analogues can be considered already at present.

FUTURE PROSPECTS IN THE SOMATOSTATIN RECEPTOR FIELD

The development of new classes of sst-subtype-selective analogues may provide us with valuable information with regard to tumour diagnosis, prognosis and prediction of SRIF analogue efficacy in the treatment of carcinoids and islet cell tumours.

Powerful α- or β-emitting isotopes coupled to somatostatin (analogues), in combination with drugs which stimulate their internalization and drugs which shorten renal accumulation of these radioligands, will potentially create the exciting new therapeutic option of internal radiotherapy for metastatic sst-positive tumours.

OTHER PEPTIDE RECEPTORS OF INTEREST FOR THE DIAGNOSIS AND THERAPY OF ISLET CELL TUMOURS AND CARCINOIDS

Other (neuro)peptide receptors, such as those for gastrin, bombesin, vasoactive intestinal polypeptide (VIP), cholecystokinin and substance P (Hennig et al, 1995; Reubi, 1995a) can be expressed by several tumours. It is, therefore, to be expected that a similar diagnostic and therapeutic development to that in the SRIF field may follow for some of these peptides and/or their analogues. Labelled (analogues of these) peptides may turn out to be successful markers for their putative receptors, not only for in vitro studies but also for in vivo tumour visualization. As a prerequisite for in vivo scintigraphy, labelled (analogues of these) peptides which are stable in the circulation and can be adequately cleared from the circulation need to be developed.

The 28-amino acid long peptide VIP is one of these promising agents for in vitro and in vivo tumour imaging. Reubi investigated 11 differentiated and six undifferentiated islet cell tumours and carcinoids by receptor autoradiography on tissue sections with [^{125}I]VIP. These results were compared with those obtained by quantitative receptor autoradiography in adjacent sections with [^{125}I-Tyr^3]octreotide. It was shown that all differentiated tumours expressed high affinity VIP receptors (VIP-Rs) and ssts. However, half of the undifferentiated tumours expressed VIP-Rs and none of these tumours expressed ssts. VIP-Rs were also expressed by 75% of pancreatic adenocarcinomas, all oesophageal squamous cell carcinomas and all colonic adenocarcinomas (Reubi, 1995b). Virgolini et al (1994) visualized nine of 10 primary carcinoid tumours and four of six carcinoid metastases by means of in vivo scintigraphy with[123]I-labelled VIP. Interestingly, VIP-Rs are also expressed in the normal gut and lymphoid tissues, but the normal tissues were not sufficiently labelled and did not interfere with the tumour imaging. Scintigraphy with [^{111}In]pentetreotide was positive in eight of nine primary carcinoid tumours and in three of six metastases. VIP-R scintigraphy was also positive in four of four primary insulinomas, whereas sst scintigraphy was positive in two of two cases. In another study, VIP-R scintigraphy was positive for one gastrinoma and negative for another gastrinoma (Virgolini et al, 1995). These studies reveal the great potential of VIP-R scintigraphy for tumour imaging in carcinoids and islet cell tumours. The functional role played by tumoral VIP-Rs needs to be elucidated, although preliminary data suggest that VIP may have proliferative actions (Reubi, 1995b).

In conclusion, VIP-R scintigraphy is a sensitive technique for the identification of islet cell tumours and carcinoids. However, like sst scintigraphy, this technique does not seem to be useful for the differential diagnosis of these tumours, as most colorectal, gastric and pancreatic adenocarcinomas are also VIP-R positive.

SUMMARY

A great number of gut endocrine tumours show high expression of receptors for neuropeptides, such as SRIF and VIP. The expression of ssts is essential for the control of hormonal hypersecretion and tumour growth by octapeptide somatostatin analogues. Five different sst subtypes, named sst_{1-5}, have been cloned and characterized. The therapeutic efficacy of the octapeptide analogues is determined by the expression of sst_2 (sst_3) and sst_5 on the tumour. In general, there is a predominant expression of sst_1 and sst_2 mRNA in gut endocrine tumours. In vivo sst scintigraphy, after injection of [^{111}In]pentetreotide, provides a useful tool for the diagnostic work-up of patients with these tumours. This technique can be used for the localization of the primary tumour(s), for the determination of the extent of metastatic spread and for the selection of potential candidates for therapy with (radio-labelled) octapeptide analogues.

Differentiated gut endocrine tumours also show a high expression of VIP-Rs. However, undifferentiated tumours show VIP-R expression to a smaller degree. In vivo scintigraphy with ^{123}I-labelled VIP is a sensitive technique for the in vivo identification of gut endocrine tumours and their metastases. The functional role of the tumoral VIP-Rs is still unclear and at present there are no known therapeutic applications for VIP-R agonists or antagonists in humans.

REFERENCES

Ahlman H, Wangberg B & Nilsson O (1993) Growth regulation in carcinoid tumors. *Endocrinology and Metabolism Clinics of North America* **22:** 889–915.
Brazeau P, Vale W, Burgus R et al (1973) Hypothalamic polypeptide that inhibits the secretion of immunoreactive pituitary growth hormone. *Science* **179:** 77–79.

Buscail L, Esteve JP, Saint-Laurent N et al (1995) Inhibition of cell proliferation by the somatostatin analogue RC-160 is mediated by somatostatin receptor subtypes SSTR2 and SSTR5 through different mechanisms. *Proceedings of the National Academy of Sciences of the USA* **92:** 1580–1584.

Evers BM, Townsend CM Jr, Upp JR et al (1991) Establishment and characterization of a human carcinoid in nude mice and effect of various agents on tumor growth. *Gastroenterology* **101:** 303–311.

van Hagen PM, Krenning EP, Kwekkeboom DJ et al (1994) Somatastatin and the immune and haematopoetic system; a review. *European Journal of Clinical Investigation* **24:** 91–99.

Hennig IM, Laissue JA, Horisberger U & Reubi JC (1995) Substance-P receptors in human primary neoplasms: tumoral and vascular localization. *International Journal of Cancer* **61:** 786–792.

Hofland LJ & Lamberts SWJ (1996) Somatostatin receptors and disease: role of receptor subtypes. In *Baillière's Clinical Endocrinology and Metabolism*, vol. 10, pp 163–176. London: Baillière Tindall.

Hofland LJ, van Koetsveld PM, Waaijers M et al (1994) Relative potencies of the somatostatin analogs octreotide, BIM-23014, and RC-160 on the inhibition of hormone release by cultured human endocrine tumor cells and normal rat anterior pituitary cells. *Endocrinology* **134:** 301–306.

Hofland LJ, van Koetsveld PM & Waaijers M et al (1995a) Internalization of the radioiodinated somatostatin analog [^{125}I-Tyr^3]octreotide by mouse and human pituitary tumor cells: increase by unlabeled octreotide. *Endocrinology* **136:** 3698–3706.

Hofland LJ, Visser-Wisselaar HA & Lamberts SW (1995b) Somatostatin analogs: clinical application in relation to human somatostatin receptor subtypes. *Biochemical Pharmacology* **50:** 287–297.

Hoyer D, Bell GI, Berelowitz M et al (1995) Classification and nomenclature of somatostatin receptors. *Trends in Pharmacological Sciences* **16:** 86–88.

Ishizuka J, Beauchamp RD, Evers BM et al (1992) Unexpected growth-stimulatory effect of somatostatin analogue on cultured human pancreatic carcinoid cells. *Biochemical and Biophysical Research Communications* **185:** 577–581.

Jamar F, Fiasse R, Leners N & Pauwels S (1995) Somatostatin receptor imaging with indium-111-pentetreotide in gastroenteropancreatic neuroendocrine tumors: safety, efficacy and impact on patient management. *Journal of Nuclear Medicine* **36:** 542–549.

Janson ET, Westlin JE, Eriksson B et al (1994) [^{111}In-DTPA-D-Phe^1]octreotide scintigraphy in patients with carcinoid tumours: the predictive value for somatostatin analogue treatment. *European Journal of Endocrinology* **131:** 577–581.

Krenning EP, Kwekkeboom DJ, Bakker WH et al (1993) Somatostatin receptor scintigraphy with [^{111}In-DTPA-D-Phe^1]- and [^{123}I-Tyr^3]-octreotide: the Rotterdam experience with more than 1000 patients. *European Journal of Nuclear Medicine* **20:** 716–731.

Krenning EP, Kwekkeboom DJ, Oei HY et al (1994a) Somatostatin-receptor scintigraphy in gastro-enteropancreatic tumors. An overview of European results. *Annals of the New York Academy of Sciences* **733:** 416–424.

Krenning EP, Kooij PP, Bakker WH et al (1994b) Radiotherapy with a radiolabeled somatostatin analogue, [^{111}In-DTPA-D-Phe^1]-octreotide. A case history. *Annals of the New York Academy of Sciences* **733:** 496–506.

Krenning EP, Kwekkeboom DJ, Pauwels S et al (1995) Somatostatin receptor scintigraphy. *Nuclear Medicine Annual* 1–50.

Kubota A, Yamada Y, Kagimoto S et al (1994) Identification of somatostatin receptor subtypes and an implication for the efficacy of somatostatin analogue SMS 201–995 in treatment of human endocrine tumors. *Journal of Clinical Investigation* **93:** 1321–1325.

Kwekkeboom DJ, Assies J, Hofland LJ et al (1993a) A case of antibody formation against octreotide visualized with ^{111}In-octreotide scintigraphy. *Clinical Endocrinology* **39:** 239–243.

Kwekkeboom DJ, Krenning EP, Bakker WH et al (1993b) Somatostatin analogue scintigraphy in carcinoid tumours. *European Journal of Nuclear Medicine* **20:** 283–292.

Lamberts SW (1988) The role of somatostatin in the regulation of anterior pituitary hormone secretion and the use of its analogs in the treatment of human pituitary tumors. *Endocrine Reviews* **9:** 417–436.

Lamberts SW, Pieters GF, Metselaar HJ et al (1988) Development of resistance to a long-acting somatostatin analogue during treatment of two patients with metastatic endocrine pancreatic tumours. *Acta Endocrinologica Copenhagen* **119:** 561–566.

Lamberts SWJ, Hofland LJ, van Koetsveld PM et al (1990) Parallel in vivo and in vitro detection of functional somatostatin receptors in human endocrine pancreatic tumors: consequences with regard to diagnosis, localization, and therapy. *Journal of Clinical Endocrinology and Metabolism* **71:** 566–574.

Lamberts SW, Krenning EP, Reubi JC (1991) The role of somatostatin and its analogs in the diagnosis and treatment of tumors. *Endocrine Reviews* **12:** 450–482.

Lamberts SW, Hofland LJ, de Herder WW et al (1993) Octreotide and related somatostatin analogs in the diagnosis and treatment of pituitary disease and somatostatin receptor scintigraphy. *Frontiers of Neuroendocrinology,* **14:** 27–55.

Lamberts SWJ, van der Lely AJ, de Herder WW & Hofland LJ (1996) Octreotide. *New England Journal of Medicine* **334:** 246–254.

Lebtahi R, Cadiot G, Sarda L et al (1994) Clinical interest of Octreoscan 111 scintigraphy in gastro-enteropancreatic tumors. *Journal of Nuclear Medicine* **35:** 96P (abstract).

Liebow C, Reilly C, Serrano M & Schally AV (1989) Somatostatin analogues inhibit growth of pancreatic cancer by stimulating tyrosine phosphatase. *Proceedings of the National Academy of Sciences of the USA* **86:** 2003–2007.

McEntee GP, Nagorney DM, Kvols LK et al (1990) Cytoreductive hepatic surgery for neuroendocrine tumors. *Surgery* **108:** 1091–1096.

Moertel CG, Kvols LK, O'Connell MJ & Rubin J (1991) Treatment of neuroendocrine carcinoma with combined etoposide and cisplatin. Evidence of major therapeutic activity in the anaplastic variants of these neoplasms. *Cancer* **68:** 227–232.

Moertel CG, Lefkopoulo M, Lipsitz S et al (1992) Streptozocin–doxorubicin, streptozocin–fluorouracil or chlorozotocin in the treatment of advanced islet-cell carcinoma. *New England Journal of Medicine* **326:** 519–523.

Moertel CG, Johnson CM, McKusick MA et al (1994) The management of patients with advanced carcinoid tumors and islet cell carcinomas. *Annals of Internal Medicine* **120:** 302–309.

Oberg K (1993) The use of chemotherapy in the management of neuroendocrine tumors. *Endocrinology and Metabolism Clinics of North America* **22:** 941–952.

Oberg K, Eriksson B & Janson ET (1994) The clinical use of interferons in the management of neuro-endocrine gastroenteropancreatic tumors. *Annals of the New York Academy of Sciences* **733:** 471–478.

Pradayrol L, Jornvall H, Mutt V & Ribet A (1980) *N*-terminally extended somatostatin: the primary structure of somatostatin-28. *FEBS Letters* **109:** 55–58.

Reisine T & Bell GI (1995) Molecular properties of somatostatin receptors. *Neuroscience* **67:** 777–790.

Reubi JC (1993) The role of peptides and their receptors as tumor markers. *Endocrinology and Metabolism Clinics of North America* **22:** 917–939.

Reubi JC (1995a) Neuropeptide receptors in health and disease: the molecular basis for in vivo imaging. *Journal of Nuclear Medicine* **36:** 1825–1835.

Reubi JC (1995b) In vitro identification of vasoactive intestinal peptide receptors in human tumors: implications for tumor imaging. *Journal of Nuclear Medicine* **36:** 1846–1853.

Reubi JC & Laissue JA (1995) Multiple actions of somatostatin in neoplastic disease. *Trends in Pharmacological Science* **16:** 110–115.

Reubi JC, Kvols LK, Waser B et al (1990) Detection of somatostatin receptors in surgical and percutaneous needle biopsy samples of carcinoids and islet cell carcinomas. *Cancer Research* **50:** 5969–5977.

Reubi JC, Krenning E, Lamberts SW & Kvols L (1992a) In vitro detection of somatostatin receptors in human tumors. *Metabolism* **41:** 104–110.

Reubi JC, Laissue J, Krenning E & Lamberts SW (1992b) Somatostatin receptors in human cancer: incidence, characteristics, functional correlates and clinical implications. *Journal of Steroid Biochemistry and Molecular Biology* **43:** 27–35.

Reubi JC, Horisberger U & Laissue J (1994a) High density of somatostatin receptors in veins surrounding human cancer tissue: role in tumor–host interaction? *International Journal of Cancer* **56:** 681–688.

Reubi JC, Laissue J, Waser B et al (1994b) Expression of somatostatin receptors in normal, inflamed, and neoplastic human gastrointestinal tissues. *Annals of the New York Academy of Sciences* **733:** 122–137.

Reubi JC, Schaer JC, Waser B & Mengod G (1994c) Expression and localization of somatostatin receptor SSTR1, SSTR2, and SSTR3 messenger RNAs in primary human tumors using in situ hybridization. *Cancer Research* **54:** 3455–3459.

Schirmer WJ, O'Dorisio TM, Schirmer TP et al (1993) Intraoperative localization of neuroendocrine tumors with 125l-TYR(3)-octreotide and a hand-held gamma-detecting probe. *Surgery* **114:** 745–751.

Srikant CB (1995) Cell cycle dependent induction of apoptosis by somatostatin analog SMS 201–995 in AtT-20 mouse pituitary cells. *Biochemical and Biophysical Research Communications* **209:** 400–406.

Srkalovic G, Cai RZ & Schally AV (1990) Evaluation of receptors for somatostatin in various tumors using different analogs. *Journal of Clinical Endocrinology and Metabolism* **70:** 661–669.

Vikic-Topic S, Raisch KP, Kvols LK & Vuk-Pavlovic S (1995) Expression of somatostatin receptor subtypes in breast carcinoma, carcinoid tumor, and renal cell carcinoma. *Journal of Clinical Endocrinology and Metabolism* **80:** 2974–2979.

Virgolini I, Raderer M, Kurtaran A et al (1994) Vasoactive intestinal peptide-receptor imaging for the localization of intestinal adenocarcinomas and endocrine tumors. *New England Journal of Medicine* **331:** 1116–1121.

Virgolini I, Kurtaran A, Raderer M et al (1995) Vasoactive intestinal peptide receptor scintigraphy. *Journal of Nuclear Medicine* **36:** 1732–1739.

3

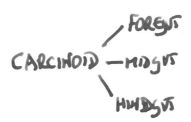

Carcinoid tumours

EVA M. TIENSUU JANSON
KJELL E. ÖBERG

In 1907 Oberndorfer introduced the term carcinoid when he described small, slowly growing tumours originating in the intestine. The carcinoid tumour was initially considered to be benign, but the true malignant potential was recognized by Pearson and Fitzgerald (1949) in their report of 140 carcinoid patients which included several patients with metastasising carcinoid tumours.

The carcinoid tumours originate from neuroendocrine cells found throughout the human body. Cells of the neuroendocrine cell system share several common features such as a positive argyrophil staining reaction and the presence of secretory granules. These tumours have traditionally been divided into three different groups according to the origin of the primary tumour (Williams and Sandler, 1963). Foregut carcinoid tumours include primaries located in the lung, stomach and proximal duodenum while midgut carcinoid tumours arise from the rest of the small intestine and colon to the mid-transverse colon. Hindgut carcinoid tumours comprise those originating from the distal part of the colon and rectum. The midgut carcinoid tumours are usually argentaffin, while the two other subgroups are usually not. The histological patterns also differ, since midgut carcinoid tumours usually grow in nests separated by connective tissue, while foregut and hindgut carcinoid tumours tend to grow in a more trabecular pattern.

While midgut carcinoid tumours are characterized by the production of high amounts of serotonin (Lembeck, 1953), foregut carcinoid tumours may also produce serotonin but adrenocorticotrophic hormone (ACTH), gastrin, calcitonin and histamine may also be present. In patients with hindgut carcinoid tumours serotonin is never produced and instead other hormones such as somatostatin and peptide YY (PYY) may be present. In all three tumour subgroups high levels of chromogranin A, PP and human chorionic gonadotrophin (HCG)-α and -β may be found (Wilander et al, 1989).

This classification based on the anatomical localization of the tumour has been questioned lately. The term carcinoid should therefore be revised in the near future to omit the present confusion. It might be kept for traditional midgut neuroendocrine tumours with the carcinoid syndrome but other tumours should be called neuroendocrine tumours attached by the primary location, for example, neuroendocrine lung, gastric, duodenal, pancreatic,

Baillière's Clinical Gastroenterology—
Vol. 10, No. 4, December 1996
ISBN 0–7020–2186–5
0950–3528/96/040589 + 13 $12.00/00

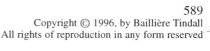

colonic and rectal tumours. The dominating hormone production may sometimes be included, for example gastrin-producing neuroendocrine duodenal tumour or ACTH-producing neuroendocrine bronchial tumour. Such a classification would certainly be helpful in communications concerning these tumours.

THE CARCINOID SYNDROME

The carcinoid syndrome may be present in patients with midgut carcinoid tumours with liver metastases, and also in some patients with foregut carcinoid tumours. Patients with hindgut carcinoid tumours do not present with this syndrome. The syndrome consists of flushes, diarrhoea, carcinoid heart disease with right-sided heart failure, bronchial constriction and elevated levels of the serotonin metabolite 5-hydroxyindoleacetic acid (5-HIAA) in the urine (Thorson et al, 1954). In some patients the syndrome may be severe enough to be potentially life threatening with extensive flushes combined with hypotension or very frequent diarrhoea, the so-called carcinoid crisis.

The cause of the different features of the carcinoid syndrome is not fully elucidated. Serotonin may be responsible for the diarrhoea (Feldman and O'Dorisio, 1986), while tachykinins such as neuropeptide K may play a role in the carcinoid flush (Norheim et al, 1986). Carcinoid heart disease with pulmonic stenosis and tricuspid regurgitation may also be induced by hormones produced by the tumour. It has been shown that the levels of both 5-HIAA and neuropeptide K are higher in patients with the carcinoid heart disease than in those without (Lundin et al, 1988). The increased fibrosis locally in the heart seems to be related to increased expression of the trans-forming growth factor (TGF)-β family of growth factors (Waltenberger et al, 1993). Future studies will have to address these possible relations.

The carcinoid flush and diarrhoea may be relieved by medical treatment. However, carcinoid heart disease in advanced stages requires open heart surgery with replacement of the affected valves. In carefully selected cases this may add several years of high quality of life to these patients.

THE DIAGNOSTIC PROCEDURE

The diagnosis and characterization of a carcinoid tumour may be divided into several parts including hormone production, histopathological evaluation, radiological examination and radionuclear investigations. Different aspects of tumour biology have also been included in the pre-treatment work-up.

Hormone production

Chromogranin A is a member of the chromogranin family consisting of at least three different water-soluble, acidic glycoproteins (Smith and

Winkler, 1967). They are stored together with peptide hormones in large dense core vesicles in endocrine and neuroendocrine cells. Increased plasma levels may be found in patients with neuroendocrine tumours (O'Connor and Deftos, 1986), and measurements of this peptide in plasma may be used as an early marker for neuroendocrine tumours including foregut, midgut and hindgut carcinoid tumours (Eriksson et al, 1990; Stridsberg et al, 1995).

The production of serotonin is characteristic for midgut carcinoid tumours, and elevated serotonin levels may be measured either in plasma or as the serotonin metabolite 5-HIAA acid in the urine (Lembeck, 1953). Although increased levels are most frequently found in patients with midgut carcinoid tumours, some patients with foregut carcinoid also display high levels. However, patients with hindgut carcinoid tumours never have elevated levels of this hormone. The level of the metabolite is usually calculated as the mean value of the excretion in two 24 hour collections of urine. Plasma serotonin is of limited value because of significant variations over time.

Neuropeptide K is a member of the tachykinin family. Increased plasma levels of this peptide are found mainly in patients with midgut carcinoid tumours and seem to be connected to the carcinoid flush (Theodorsson-Norheim et al, 1985). During flush provocation with pentagastrin neuropeptide K levels in plasma increase in patients experiencing a carcinoid flush, and this test may be used as an early indicator of carcinoid disease in patients with normal basal levels (Norheim et al, 1986). Another tachykinin, substance P, may also be elevated in patients with midgut carcinoid tumours, but is not correlated with the carcinoid flush (Feldman and O'Dorisio, 1986).

Levels of the α and β subunits of HCG may be increased in serum in patients with carcinoid tumours. High levels of the α subunit are often found in patients with hindgut and foregut carcinoid tumours, while both the α and the β subunit may be increased in midgut carcinoid patients. However, the increase is usually not impressive in midgut carcinoid patients, and it is therefore seldomly used for monitoring.

The frequency of elevated levels of different hormones in a study including 301 carcinoid patients is indicated in Table 1 (Tiensuu Janson, 1995).

Table 1. Percentage of patients with elevated levels of hormones in the different subgroups of patients.

Tumour marker	Tumour		
	Foregut	Midgut	Hindgut
U-5-HIAA	31%	76%	0%
P-chromogranin	79%	87%	100%
P-neuropeptide K	9%	46%	0%
HCG-α	35%	11%	100%
HCG-β	0%	8%	0%

Histopathology

All carcinoid tumours are stained positive with the argyrophil stain of Grimelius and immunohistochemically using chromogranin A antibodies. All midgut carcinoid tumours are also stained positive with the argentaffin stain of Masson (Wilander et al, 1989) while foregut and hindgut carcinoid tumours are argentaffin negative. The growth pattern may also differ between the three groups of carcinoid tumours as indicated above.

In the last few years other histopathological features of carcinoid tumours have been investigated. Immunohistochemistry with Ki-67 antibodies directed towards a proliferation antigen has rendered some interesting results. It has been shown that low proliferation activity in tumour specimens obtained from patients with midgut carcinoid tumours is correlated with a longer survival of the patient (Chaudhry et al, 1992). The same finding has been observed in patients with bronchopulmonary carcinoid tumours (Costes et al, 1995). It has also been suggested that the presence of one of the splice variants of CD44 in a primary tumour may indicate a tendency towards a more malignant form and promote a metastatic behaviour (Gunthert et al, 1991). Larger molecular forms of CD44 are found in patients with foregut carcinoid tumours (Chaudhry et al, 1994).

Radiological examination

In the staging procedure of patients with carcinoid tumours computerized tomography (CT), magnetic resonance imaging (MRI) and ultrasonography are most frequently used. Liver metastases are the most common finding. When present, mesenteric metastases may produce a typical finding with a tumour mass surrounded by linear, radiating soft tissue spokes (Dudiak et al, 1989). If the site of the primary tumour is unclear, further examinations including arteriography may be of value but this has been replaced by somatostatin receptor scintigraphy (see below). In patients with symptoms of intestinal obstruction a barium enema may indicate the presence of a tumour in the small intestine.

Radionuclear investigations

During the last few years new methods based on tumour-seeking substances labelled with radioactive compounds have become frequently used in the diagnostic procedure as well as for biological characterization of neuroendocrine tumours.

Positron emission tomography (PET) is a recently developed technique which may be used for the localization of carcinoid tumours. ^{11}C-labelled 5-hydroxitryptophan (HTP) (a precursor of the serotonin synthesis) is taken up by the carcinoid tumour. The current detection limit is a tumour size of about 5 mm. It is as sensitive as somatostatin receptor scintigraphy and shows higher sensitivity than a CT-scan (Eriksson et al, unpublished). As well as giving the tumour localization it also provides information about tumour metabolism and can demonstrate effects of various treatments. By labelling other tracer substances one can study various aspects of tumour biology in vivo in the patient.

It is well established that carcinoid tumours have a high expression of somatostain receptors. More than 90% of patients with midgut carcinoid tumours express somatostatin receptors detected by autoradiography techniques with iodinated somatostatin analogues as ligands, while the somatostatin receptor expression in foregut carcinoid tumours is less frequent (Reubi et al, 1990). There seems to be a correlation between in vitro detection of somatostatin receptors and the response to somatostatin analogue treatment.

Until now five different subtypes of somatostatin receptors have been cloned. We know that somatostatin receptor subtype 2 binds the somatostatin analogues used in the clinic with high affinity. Subtypes 3 and 5 have an intermediate affinity, while subtypes 1 and 4 have low affinity for the available somatostatin analogues (Reisine and Bell, 1995).

A technique using the somatostatin analogue octreotide, labelled with radioactive indium, to visualize neuroendocrine tumours has been developed (Bakker et al, 1991). The [^{111}In-DTPA-D-Phe^1]octreotide (Octreoscan®) is injected intravenously and the patient is examined with a γ camera on the following day. This investigation provides information on the somatostatin receptor status of the patient's tumours, and also gives a whole-body examination with the chance to identify tumour lesions outside the abdomen. The usefulness of this imaging technique for patients with carcinoid tumours is now established (Kwekkeboom et al, 1993) (Figure 1).

It has been shown that the somatostatin receptor status of the tumour detected by somatostatin receptor scintigraphy may be used to predict which patients may respond with a decrease in hormone levels following medical treatment with a somatostatin analogue (Tiensuu Janson et al, 1994). However, about 20% of patients with tracer uptake in tumour lesions do not respond to such treatment. The reason for this may be that the tracer can bind to different subtypes of the somatostatin receptor, while only one of the subtypes, subtype 2, is known to inhibit hormone release. A correlation between the presence of somatostatin receptor subtype 2 mRNA expression and response to somatostatin analogue treatment has been found in single patients (Kubota et al, 1994; Tiensuu Janson et al, 1996). However, a heterogeneous expression within the same tumour may also explain why patients with tracer uptake in tumour lesions fail to respond to somatostatin analogue treatment (Reubi et al, 1994).

In the future somatostatin analogues labelled with ^{111}In or other radioactive substances may be used to treat patients with somatostatin receptor positive tumours.

Recently, vasoactive intestinal peptide (VIP) receptor scintigraphy was introduced as another method for imaging gastrointestinal tumours (Virgolini et al, 1994). Nine out of 10 patients with carcinoid tumours showed positive scans with this investigation. However, VIP receptors are also present in adenocarcinomas and 10 out of 10 colorectal carcinomas were visualized, whereas colorectal carcinomas usually are negative on Octreoscan®.

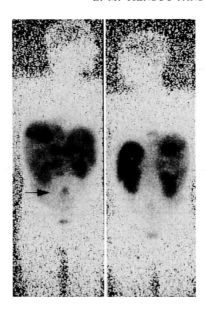

Figure 1. [¹¹¹In-DTPA-D-Phe¹]octreotide scintigraphy. Frontal view to the left and dorsal view to the right, showing a patient with a midgut carcinoid tumour. Multiple liver metastases are seen. A mesenterial metastasis is indicated by an arrow. Normal uptake in the spleen and kidneys is seen on the dorsal view. The investigation was performed at the Department of Oncology, Nuclear Section, University Hospital, Uppsala, Sweden.

Another interesting compound is [*m*-¹³¹I]iodobenzylguanidine ([¹³¹I]MIBG) which is used to detect and treat pheochromocytomas and neuroblastomas. [¹³¹I]MIBG has been tried in patients with carcinoid tumours and may accumulate in tumour lesions. However, the therapeutic value of this radiopharmaceutical in carcinoid patients has to be further investigated (Hoefnagel et al, 1986; Watanabe et al, 1995).

FEATURES OF THE DIFFERENT CARCINOID TUMOUR SUBGROUPS

Foregut tumours

Williams and Azzopardi (1960) described bronchial carcinoid tumours as a group of tumours related to carcinoid tumours originating in the gut. The bronchial carcinoid tumours seem to affect patients at a slightly earlier age than the other groups of carcinoid tumours. Bronchial carcinoid tumours may, apart from serotonin, produce other hormones such as ACTH and growth hormone releasing hormone (GHRH). These give rise to very specific symptoms including Cushing's syndrome and acromegaly. Those tumours that have serotonin production may present a carcinoid syndrome.

Some patients' tumours produce histamine and those patients may experience the histamine flush which is a bright-red flush accompanied by a swelling of the face and lacrimation.

Although there are benign bronchial carcinoid tumours, about 35–40% are malignant and these tend to have a high proliferation rate with a large proportion of cells staining positive for Ki-67. Malignant bronchial carcinoid tumours often develop metastases outside the liver. Cutaneous metastases, as well as metastases to the central nervous system and bone, are frequently seen early in the course of the disease (Grahame-Smith, 1972). About 30% of foregut carcinoid patients do not express somatostatin receptors as detected by [^{111}In-DTPA-D-Phe^1]octreotide scintigraphy, and this feature may be a bad prognostic factor (Reubi et al, 1990; Tiensuu Janson et al, 1994).

Thymic carcinoid tumours are very rare. These tumours may also produce hormones other than serotonin, for instance ACTH and calcitonin. They tend to have local recurrences giving rise to symptoms due to compression of the large vessels and trachea. Spread of the disease is related to bad prognosis and short survival.

Carcinoid tumours originating in the stomach

Gastric carcinoids have been identified in two main variants.

Type I (ECL-oma) originates from the mucosal enterochromaffin-like cells which can synthesize and store histamine. These tumours are localized in the gastric fundus and body of the stomach and are mostly multiple and associated with type A chronic atrophic gastritis, achlorhydria and often pernicious anaemia. They are accompanied by antral G cell hyperplasia. On histopathological examination different stages of ECL cell hyperplasia are noticed from small nests of ECL cells via linear hyperplasia to established polyps. The pathogenesis of these tumours is claimed to be the trophic effect of the hypergastrinaemia on ECL cells. Another cause of hypergastrinaemia leading to gastrin-dependent carcinoids in the stomach is the Zollinger–Ellison syndrome, with or without association with multiple endocrine neoplasia type 1 (MEN 1). ECL-omas related to chronic atrophic gastritis type A are rarely malignant, less than 1%, whereas tumours related to MEN 1 metastasize in 10–20% of cases (Rindi et al, 1993).

Type II or 'mixed cellular composition' gastric carcinoid tumour is not associated with hypergastrinaemia. It usually appears as a single large neoplasm with high malignant potential in patients without type A chronic atrophic gastritis, pernicious anaemia or the Zollinger–Ellison syndrome. They often present mastastases at the time of diagnosis. This type might also include some neuroendocrine carcinomas and mixed endocrine and exocrine tumours (Solcia et al, 1989).

An important diagnostic procedure in these patients is gastroscopy with subsequent histopathology. Biochemically they can all be diagnosed by measurements of chromogranin A, and measurement of histamine metabolites in the urine may be helpful in patients with type I carcinoid tumours.

In the group of foregut tumours, duodenal carcinoids are also included. These tumours might be either solitary or multiple and secrete either gastrin or somatostatin. A majority of these tumours are related to MEN 1 and sometimes also to von Recklinghausen's disease.

Midgut tumours

Midgut carcinoid tumours may be looked on as two different entities. The appendix carcinoid tumours are usually benign and discovered en passant at appendectomy (Moertel, 1987). These usually benign tumours constitute about 80% of all midgut carcinoid tumours. Appendix carcinoid tumours are mostly found at the tip of the appendix, a site which seldomly gives rise to intestinal obstruction. In a few cases the appendix carcinoid originates at the base, and these tumours may have to be removed because of intestinal obstruction. These may also show tumour biology similar to other midgut carcinoids. Tumours >2 cm in diameter tend to metastasize, and more extensive surgery should then be performed. The mucus-producing carcinoid tumours (Goblet cell carcinoid) which may arise in the appendix or caecum are usually malignant and may present a therapeutic challenge.

Midgut carcinoid tumours located outside the appendix have a greater potential for developing metastases and producing the carcinoid syndrome (Moertel et al, 1961). The most frequently found location is in the distal ileum or caecum. Some patients with midgut carcinoid tumours present with total intestinal obstruction, leading to acute operation. If all tumours can be removed there is a good chance that the patient may be cured. However, even though metastases are not found at the time of diagnosis, they may develop and become clinically overt after several years (Moertel, 1987).

Patients with the carcinoid syndrome have metastases to local lymph nodes and to the liver already at diagnosis. In these patients high levels of 5-HIAA are found in the urine. The diagnosis may become clear during an investigation owing to frequent diarrhoea or cutaneous flushes. In a few cases the diagnosis is suspected as a result of a right-sided heart failure with involvement of the tricuspid and pulmonic valves.

Hindgut tumours

The hindgut carcinoid tumours may be divided into rectal and colonic, the vast majority of which are rectal carcinoid tumours. About 5–40% of rectal carcinoid tumours are malignant (Mani et al, 1994). Colonic carcinoid tumours are rare and usually diagnosed at a late stage (Spread et al, 1994). The hormone content in hindgut carcinoid tumours is diverse and rarely includes serotonin. Instead PP, PYY and somatostatin may be present in the tumour cells (Wilander et al, 1989). These patients do usually not suffer from symptoms due to hormone production but merely from intestinal obstruction, bleeding or a large abdominal mass.

SURVIVAL AND PROGNOSIS

In the beginning of the 20th century, carcinoid tumours were considered to be benign. Today we know that in the midgut region this is true only of the small appendiceal carcinoid tumours, while carcinoid tumours originating in other locations very well may be malignant. It has been proposed that patients operated for ileal midgut carcinoid tumours with removal of the primary tumour and regional lymph nodes may be cured of the disease. However, it has been reported that the median duration to recurrence for these patients in general is about 3–4 years but may be as long as 16 years (Moertel, 1987). Thus, there is an open question as to whether these patients should receive adjuvant therapy for some time after the operation to prevent late recurrences.

The 5-year survival in patients with liver metastases of midgut carcinoid tumours has been reported to be between 38% (Zeitels et al, 1982) and 25% (McDermott et al, 1994), while the 5-year survival in patients with lymph node metastases is about 43% (McDermott et al, 1994) and 59% (Zeitels et al, 1982). In a study from our clinic (Norheim et al, 1987) the 5-year survival in patients with malignant carcinoid tumours was 65%. Recent data show that the 5-year survival in midgut carcinoid patients with lymph node metastases is 73%, in patients with one to four liver metastases 79% and in patients with five or more liver metastases 47% (Tiensuu Janson, 1995). Thus, patients with few liver metastases have a long life expectancy and it is important to treat these patients with the best medical options available, since they have many years ahead and therefore symptomatic control is of great importance. Those with massive liver involvement should receive a more aggressive treatment since the prognosis is worse.

Since carcinoid tumours may look the same on histopathology but may behave very differently in the clinic it is of great interest to find factors that may help the clinician to select patients that should receive a more aggressive treatment and those whose tumours will have a slow progression over time. In a study by Greenberg et al (1987) it was found that increasing age, advanced stage, tumours located in the large bowel and the occurrence of another malignancy were associated with an increased risk of death in gastrointestinal carcinoid tumours. However, in another study male gender emerged as a predictive factor for death from any cause, while the presence of metastases increased the risk of fatal outcome caused by the tumour (McDermott et al 1994) and age did not affect survival.

Identification of high proliferation by Ki-67 may help to find patients with rapidly growing tumours, but there are also other indicators of bad prognosis. Bad prognostic factors for midgut carcinoid patients are high levels of U-5-HIAA, neuropeptide K and chromogranin A in plasma. In a multivariate analysis including 71 patients plasma chromogranin A >5000 µg/l was found to be an independent factor of bad prognosis in patients with malignant carcinoid tumours and the median survival was significantly shorter in these patients (Figure 2). The median survival was also shorter in patients with high levels of U-5-HIAA and neuropeptide K (Table 2) (Tiensuu Janson, 1995).

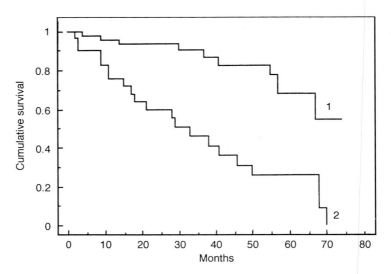

Figure 2. Survival curve indicating the cumulative survival in midgut carcinoid patients. There is a significant ($P < 0.01$) difference in survival between patients with plasma chromogranin levels <5000 µg/l (75 nmol/l) (curve 1) and those with higher levels (curve 2).

Table 2. Median survival in midgut carcinoid patients with respect to hormone levels.

Tumour marker	Median survival	P value
U-5-HIAA (<300 µmol/24 hours)	72 months	
U-5-HIAA (>300 µmol/24 hours)	45 months	<0.01
P-chromogranin (<5000 µg/l)	>57 months	
P-chromogranin (<5000 µg/l)	33 months	<0.01
P-neuropeptide K (<16 pmol/l)	72 months	
P-neuropeptide K (>16 pmol/l)	55 months	<0.05

Bronchial carcinoid tumours may be benign, but about 35–40% develop metastases. In a population-based study, stage at diagnosis was a strong determinant of survival (Greenberg et al, 1987). In this study 65% of the patients had only localized disease at diagnosis and the 5-year survival in this group was about 97%. However, patients with distant metastases at diagnosis had a risk of death that was 20 times higher than those with local disease, and the 5-year survival in this group with widespread disease was only about 42%. Stage and surgery were found to be independent predictors of death in the multivariate analysis.

In a recent study from our institution the survival for type 1 and type 2 gastric carcinoids is quite different. Nine patients with type 1 carcinoids were all alive after 18 years of observation, whereas six patients with type 2 were dead within 2 years from diagnosis (unpublished observation).

In patients with hindgut carcinoid tumours those appearing in the rectum are usually benign with only about 20% presenting with local or distant

1984). Numerous studies demonstrate that hypergastrinaemic effects on the ECL cells lead to hypergastrinaemically-induced gastric carcinoid tumours (ECLomas) (Hakanson et al, 1984; Creutzfeldt, 1988; Helander and Bordi, 1995; Willems, 1995). Studies in animals such as the rat demonstrate that hypergastrinaemia induces ECL hypertrophy within days and hyperplasia within weeks (Hakanson et al, 1984; Helander and Bordi, 1995; Willems, 1995). It has been proposed that a hyperplasia–neoplasia sequence occurs with first simple hyperplasia, followed by linear hyperplasia, micronodular hyperplasia, adenomatoid hyperplasia, dysplasia (pre-carcinoid), and finally the carcinoid stage (Solcia et al, 1988; Maton and Dayal, 1991; Jensen and Dayal, 1992). This progression is much more advanced in patients with ZES with MEN 1 than patients with ZES without MEN 1 (Lehy et al, 1992). In patients without MEN 1, fundic argyrophilic cells show a normal pattern in 16%, a diffuse pattern in 71%, and a linear pattern in 13% (Lehy et al, 1992), whereas, in patients with ZES and MEN 1, diffuse hyperplasia occurred in 53% and linear hyperplasia in 47% and 36% had invasive carcinoids (Lehy et al, 1992; Ruszniewski et al, 1993a). It had been noted earlier in studies of omeprazole-induced hypergastrin-aemia in rats that submucosal invasion could be found in 19% of animals treated long term (Havu, 1986; Helander and Bordi, 1995). Gastric

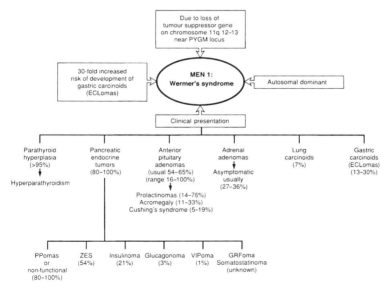

Figure 3. MEN 1 syndrome. This autosomal dominant syndrome occurs in 20–25% of patients with ZES (Jensen and Gardner, 1993; Mignon et al, 1995b) and recent linkage analysis demonstrates the genetic defect is on chromosome 11q12–13 near the skeletal muscle glycogen phosphorylase locus (PYGM) (Norton et al, 1993; Skogseid and Oberg, 1995). It is characterized by hyperplasia or tumours of multiple endocrine organs with the following relative frequency: parathyroid > pancreas > pituitary > adrenal > gastric ECL cells > lung. Patients with MEN 1 with ZES have a marked increased risk of developing gastric carcinoid tumours compared with patients without MEN 1 (Solcia et al, 1989, 1990; Jensen 1993).

carcinoids develop in 5% of patients with pernicious anaemia and 3% with ZES (Maton and Dayal, 1991; Jensen and Dayal, 1992). In ZES, more than 95% of the gastric carcinoids occur in patients with MEN 1 with ZES (Solcia et al, 1986; Frucht et al, 1991; Jensen, 1993). In one study (Frucht et al, 1991), of the 15 reported cases of gastric carcinoids in patients with ZES, MEN 1 was present in 14 patients. In two series 13% of patients with ZES and MEN 1 had a gastric carcinoid tumour in one study (Jensen, 1993) and 30% in another study (Lehy et al, 1992), whereas 0.6% (Jensen, 1993) and 0% (Lehy et al, 1992) had a gastric carcinoid tumour in the patients with MEN 1. Recent studies (Cadiot et al, 1993; Debelenko et al, 1996) demonstrate that the gastric carcinoid tumours that develop in patients with MEN 1 are due to loss of heterozygosity on chromosome 11q12 in the area in which the defect that causes MEN 1 is thought to occur (Skogseid and Oberg, 1995; Weber and Jensen, 1996) (Figure 3).

CLINICAL FEATURES

General

ZES is slightly more common in males (60%); the mean age at the onset of symptoms is approximately 50 years with a range of 7–90 years (Jensen and Gardner, 1993). From 20% to 25% of patients have the MEN 1 syndrome (Jensen and Gardner, 1993; Mignon et al, 1995b).

In most patients the initial symptoms as well as the persisting symptoms are due to the effects of gastric acid hypersecretion (Jensen et al, 1983b; Jensen and Gardner, 1993; Mignon et al, 1995b). Only late in the course of the disease in patients with general metastatic disease are the symptoms caused by the gastrinoma itself (Jensen et al, 1983b; Jensen and Gardner, 1993). Abdominal pain primarily due to peptic ulcer disease or reflux oesophagitis is the most common symptom, occurring in >75% of patients in series either alone or in combination with diarrhoea. The abdominal pain in patients with ZES generally is clinically indistinguishable from that which occurs in patients with idiopathic peptic ulcer disease (Jensen et al, 1983b; Jensen and Gardner, 1993). In early studies diarrhoea was reported in only 7% of cases alone, occurring with abdominal pain in 30%, and oesophageal symptoms alone were reported in 0–6% of patients (Ellison and Wilson, 1964; Jensen and Gardner, 1993). More recently, diarrhoea and oesophageal disease are being increasingly recognized (Jensen and Gardner, 1993; Mignon et al, 1995b). Oesophageal symptoms are now frequently described with 31% having pyrosis and/or dysphagia as the initial symptom in one recent large series, and 45–60% of patients having oesophageal symptoms and/or oesophageal lesions at presentation (Miller et al, 1990; Jensen and Gardner, 1993; Mignon et al, 1995b). Diarrhoea is frequently the sole presenting feature and in several recent studies it is the second most common clinical feature occurring alone in 9–20% of patients alone or with abdominal pain in 49–65% (Jensen and Gardner, 1993; Mignon et al, 1995b). Patients with ZES continue to present with complications of peptic ulcer disease (Table 1) such as recurrent upper gastro-intestinal (UGI) bleeding, persistent nausea and vomiting or intestinal per-foration, which are reported to occur in 10%, 31% and 7% of patients in recent studies (Waxman et al, 1991; Jensen and Maton, 1992).

In early studies 93% of patients with ZES had a peptic ulcer, and in 14–52% the ulcers were multiple or in unusual locations (Jensen and Gardner, 1993). Whereas atypical ulcers, multiple ulcers or ulcers in unusual locations should still suggest the diagnosis (Table 1), today most patients with ZES have a typical solitary duodenal ulcer and 18–25% have no ulcer at the time of diagnosis (Jensen et al, 1983b; Jensen and Gardner, 1993).

Table 1. Clinical and laboratory conditions that should lead to suspicion of Zollinger–Ellison syndrome.

A. Clinical features
  1. In a patient with a duodenal ulcer
    a. Presence of diarrhoea
    b. No *H. pylori* present
    c. Failure to heal with treatment of the *H. pylori* or with histamine H_2-receptor antagonists
    d. Presence of a pancreatic tumour
    e. Nephrolithiases or endocrinopathies
  2. Severe peptic ulcer disease leading to a complication (perforation, intractability, bleeding)
  3. Multiple duodenal ulcers or ulcers in unusual locations
  4. Severe or resistant peptic oesophageal disease
  5. Chronic secretory diarrhoea
  6. Family history of nephrolithiasis or endocrinopathies, peptic ulcer disease or MEN 1

B. Laboratory features in a patient with peptic ulcer disease that should suggest ZES
  1. Hypergastrinaemia
  2. Hypercalcaemia
  3. Endocrinopathy
  4. Prominent gastric folds on UGI X-ray or at endoscopy
  5. Lack of *H. pylori*
  6. Gastric acid hypersecretion

Patients with ZES with MEN 1

MEN 1 is an autosomal dominant disease characterized by hyperplasia or tumours of multiple endocrine organs, particularly the parathyroid glands, pancreas, pituitary and, to a lesser degree, the adrenal gland, lung and gastric mucosa (Jensen and Gardner, 1993; Metz et al, 1994) (Figure 3).

Primary hyperparathyroidism causing hypercalcaemia is the most common clinical abnormality in patients with MEN 1, occurring in 95–98% (Jensen and Gardner, 1993; Metz et al, 1994; Skogseid and Öberg, 1995) (Figure 3). PETs occur in 80–100% of patients, with non-functional tumours or pancreatic polypeptide-producing tumours (PPomas) being the most common and functional PETs developing in approximately 80% of patients (Jensen and Gardner, 1993; Metz et al, 1994). Gastrinomas are the most common functional PET, occurring in 54% of patients, whereas insulinomas occur in 21%, glucagonomas in 3%, and VIPomas in 1% (Jensen and Gardner, 1993; Metz et al, 1994). Pituitary adenomas occur in

16–100% of patients and may cause symptoms as a result of local encroachment or hormone release. In various studies 41–76% are prolactinomas, 11–33% are associated with acromegaly, and Cushing's syndrome develops in 5–19% (Maton et al, 1986; Norton et al, 1993; Metz et al, 1994) (Figure 3).

Patients with ZES and MEN 1 are clinically different from patients with the sporadic form of ZES in that they characteristically present at an early age (43 versus 48 years in one study) (Mignon et al, 1995b), most patients have hyperparathyroidism or pituitary disease at the time of the presentation of the ZES, and the presence of the hypercalcaemia can make it more difficult to control the gastric acid hypersecretion (Norton et al, 1987; Jensen and Gardner, 1993; Metz et al, 1994). Patients with MEN 1 with ZES also differ from those without MEN 1 in the role of surgical resection in treatment, the percentage with the aggressive form of the disease and long-term survival in some studies (Jensen and Gardner, 1993; Weber and Jensen, 1996), each of which will be discussed in later sections related to these areas.

DIAGNOSIS AND DIFFERENTIAL DIAGNOSIS

Features that should suggest ZES

There continues to be a mean delay from the onset of ZES to its diagnosis of 3–6 years in most series (Jensen and Gardner, 1993). This delay occurs principally because ZES is an uncommon condition (one to three new cases per million population per year) which is not considered, especially early in its course, because it mimics common conditions such as peptic ulcer disease which has >1000-fold incidence at 230 new cases per 100 000 population per year and reflux oesophagitis which occurs in 3–4% of the population. In addition, most patients with ZES present with duodenal ulcer disease which is clinically and endoscopically indistinguishable from a peptic ulcer in a patient with idiopathic peptic disease. However, there are certain clinical and laboratory features (Table 1) that should suggest ZES. ZES should be especially suspected in a patient with peptic ulcer disease (PUD) who also has diarrhoea. Diarrhoea is currently rarely seen in patients with idiopathic PUD now that antacids are not used. In various studies 30–65% of patients with ZES present with diarrhoea and in 7–20% of patients the diarrhoea is the main symptom (Jensen and Gardner, 1993; Mignon et al, 1995b). Therefore, in a patient with chronic diarrhoea that persists during fasting or decreases with gastric acid antisecretory treatment, ZES should be suspected. ZES should also be suspected if *Helicobacter pylori* is not present in a patient with duodenal ulcer disease because *H. pylori* is present in 90–98% of idiopathic duodenal ulcers, but in <50% of patients with ZES (Metz et al, 1995; Weber et al, 1995a) (Table 1). Conversely, >90% of idiopathic PUD heals with eradication of *H. pylori* or with histamine H_2-receptor antagonist treatment, and therefore a failure to heal a duodenal ulcer with these treatments should lead to a suspicion of

ZES. The PUD in patients with ZES is frequently more severe than routine PUD; therefore, any patient with multiple refractory disease or complications of PUD including refractory reflux symptoms or oesophageal strictures, ulcers or ulcers in unusual locations, should be suspected of having ZES (Jensen and Gardner, 1993; Weber et al, 1995a) (Table 1). In any patient with PUD found to have hypergastrinaemia, ZES should be entertained. Prominent gastric folds are uncommon in patients with routine PUD and, if these are found by UGI X-ray studies or UGI endoscopy, ZES should be suspected. Any patient with PUD with a pancreatic tumour, especially if it is endocrine in origin, should be considered as possibly having ZES. Lastly, 20–25% of patients with ZES have MEN 1 with the presence of other endocrinopathies, a family history of other endocrinopathies, particularly nephrolithiasis, hypercalcaemia or other laboratory data suggesting endocrinopathies and, therefore, their occurrence in a patient with PUD should raise the possibility of ZES (Table 1, Figure 3).

Diagnosis and differential diagnosis of ZES

When the diagnosis of ZES is suspected, fasting serum gastrin level and the gastric pH should be measured to determine whether the patient may have ZES (Wolfe and Jensen, 1987; Jensen and Gardner, 1993; Weber et al, 1995a). Usually, only the fasting gastrin level is measured initially. Fasting serum gastrin levels were reported to be elevated in >98% of patients with ZES, especially if drawn on at least two separate occasions (Jensen and Gardner, 1993). Recently (Jais and Mignon, 1995; Zimmer et al, 1995) patients with ZES with normal fasting gastrins at presentation have been described, constituting 17% of the patients in one series (Jais and Mignon, 1995). Many of these patients, however, had positive secretin provocative tests. In most series (Jensen and Gardner, 1993), >90% of patients with ZES at presentation will have an elevated fasting serum gastrin, and therefore this test remains the best single initial screening study. If the fasting serum gastrin level is elevated, then it should be repeated and gastric fluid pH measured at the same time. If the fasting gastrin concentration remains elevated and the gastric fluid has a pH <2.5, then the patient may have ZES. If the pH is >2.5 it is very unlikely that the hypergastrinaemia is due to ZES and it is likely to be due to one of the other causes of hypochlorhydria or achlorhydria listed in Table 2. Drug-induced hypergastrinaemia can be particularly difficult to differentiate from ZES and is now a frequent cause of hypergastrinaemia. With the increased use of long-acting acid suppressant agents such as the H^+–K^+-ATPase inhibitors (omeprazole and lansoprazole), this is becoming an increasing problem. In recent studies 80–100% of patients with idiopathic reflux disease treated long term with omeprazole develop hypergastrinaemia and in some studies 20% of patients develop a serum gastrin level increase to more than five times the normal level (Jansen et al, 1990; Lamberts et al, 1993). Therefore, if the patient is taking these antisecretory drugs, the hypergastrinaemia could be either drug induced or caused by a gastric acid hypersecretory state that caused the symptoms that led to the patient being treated with these drugs. To distinguish between

Table 2. Causes of chronic hypergastrinaemia.

A. Associated with gastric acid hyposecretion–achlorhydria
  1. Pernicious anaemia–atrophic gastritis
  2. Treatment with potent gastric acid antisecretory agents (especially with H^+–K^+-ATPase inhibitors: omeprazole, lansoprazole)
  3. Chronic renal failure (common)
  4. *H. pylori* infection
  5. Post-gastric acid-reducing surgery
B. Associated with gastric acid hypersecretion
  1. *H. pylori* infection
  2. Gastric outlet obstruction
  3. Antral G-cell hyperfunction–hyperplasia
  4. Chronic renal failure (rare)
  5. Retained gastric antrum syndrome
  6. Short-bowel syndrome
  7. ZES

these two possibilities, H^+–K^+-ATPase inhibitors need to be stopped for at least 7 days and histamine H_2-blockers for at least 30 hours prior to the determination of gastric pH. If the gastric pH fluid is <2.5 and the serum gastrin level is >1000 pg/ml (normal <100 pg/ml), the patient almost certainly has ZES if the possibility of the retained gastric antrum syndrome (see below) can be excluded. In one large study 30% of patients with ZES fall into this category (Jensen, 1993). A number of conditions can cause moderate elevations of serum gastrin levels (101–999 pg/ml, normal <100 pg/ml) and a gastric pH <2.5 (Table 2) and ZES has to be distinguished from these conditions. Seventy per cent of patients fall into this range with their fasting gastrin levels between 101 and 999 pg/ml (Jensen, 1993).

In patients in whom ZES is strongly suspected but fasting gastrin levels are normal or in patients with moderate serum gastrin elevations (101–999 pg/ml) with the gastric fluid pH <2.5, a gastric analysis as well as a secretin test should be performed to measure BAO (Weber et al, 1995a; Mignon et al, 1995b).

Most patients with ZES have a BAO >15 mEq/hour for patients without previous acid-reducing surgery and >5 mEq/hour for those with previous acid-reducing surgery (Jensen and Maton, 1992; Jensen and Gardner, 1993). These criteria will include 66–99% of patients with ZES and exclude 90% of patients with duodenal ulcer disease (Mignon et al, 1995b; Weber et al, 1995a). These criteria, unfortunately, are not specific for ZES and can occur in a number of conditions listed in Table 2 associated with gastric acid hypersecretion. To distinguish ZES from these other conditions, a secretin provocative test should be performed by measuring fasting gastrin levels before and 2, 5, 10 and 20 min after the intravenous bolus injection of secretin (2 clinical units/kg). A post-secretin gastrin level ≥200 pg/ml above the pre-injection serum gastrin level is a positive response and this will occur in 87% of patients with ZES (Frucht et al, 1989b). The secretin provocative test has no reported false-positive responses in patients that are not achlorhydric (Frucht et al, 1989b). One-third of the 13% of patients with ZES with a negative secretin test will have a positive calcium infusion test (Frucht et al, 1989b) and many of the remainder will have positive tumour imaging studies supporting a diagnosis of ZES. If a patient has a negative secretin test and fits the other criteria for ZES, or ZES is strongly suspected but has *H. pylori*, then the *H. pylori* should be treated and the patient reassessed post-eradication of the *H. pylori*. Recent reports describe such patients who did not have ZES but had hypergastrinaemia and hyperchlorhydria, which was due to the *H. pylori* infection (el-Omar et al, 1995; Metz et al, 1995).

The diagnosis of MEN 1 with ZES

Whether or not a patient with ZES had MEN 1, until recently, was not generally thought difficult to determine (Wolfe and Jensen, 1987; Jensen and Gardner, 1993; Metz et al, 1994; Weber et al, 1995a). This occurred because it was generally accepted that 95–98% of patients with ZES as part of the MEN 1 syndrome (Figure 3) had already developed hyperparathyroidism or pituitary disease prior to the ZES. Therefore, by measuring serum calcium levels and plasma PTH levels, or evaluating the pituitary at the time of the diagnosis of ZES, it would be easy to establish whether it was occurring as part of the MEN 1 syndrome (Figure 3). Recent studies show that patients with MEN 1 can initially present solely with a PET or ZES, and therefore it may be difficult to distinguish patients with ZES with or without MEN 1 (Shepherd et al, 1993; Benya et al, 1994). In one recent study (Benya et al, 1994), one-third of the 28 patients with MEN 1 and ZES initially presented with ZES and only developed hyperparathyroidism or pituitary dysfunction later in the disease course. Despite serial serum calcium levels, plasma PTH levels and pituitary studies, in this study (Benya et al, 1994) in one-third of patients with ZES, the diagnosis of MEN 1 was not established until 12–264 months after the diagnosis of ZES (Benya et al, 1994). These data led to the suggestion (Benya et al, 1994) that, when specific genetic tests for MEN 1 become available, all patients with ZES should be examined because of the effect of the diagnosis of MEN 1 on the approach to treatment and the need for family screening.

TREATMENT

Treatment of the gastric acid hypersecretion

General

The first goal in the management of patients with ZES is to control the gastric acid hypersecretion. The gastric acid secretion should be controlled as soon as the diagnosis is suspected and even before the diagnosis is completely established if the patient is acutely ill because complications can develop rapidly in these patients owing to the massive acid hypersecretion that is frequently present.

Gastric acid hypersecretion should be treated medically in all patients with ZES except for the small percentage ($<1\%$) who cannot or will not take oral gastric acid antisecretory agents (Jensen and Gardner, 1993; Jensen and Fraker, 1994; Norton 1994; Metz and Jensen, 1995; Weber et al, 1995a). The acid antisecretory drugs of choice are now the H^+–K^+-ATPase inhibitors, either omeprazole or lansoprazole (Metz and Jensen, 1995; Weber et al, 1995a). These agents are longer acting than the histamine H_2-receptor antagonists, with the result that once or twice a day dosing is possible in almost every patient (Frucht et al, 1991; Jensen and Gardner, 1993; Metz and Jensen, 1995). Omeprazole and lansoprazole have similar long durations of action ($t_{0.5} = 35$ hours) and appear indistinguishable in their kinetics of action in ZES (Metz et al, 1993c,d; Metz and Jensen, 1995). There is, however, much more experience with omeprazole than lansoprazole and it has been used over a much longer period of time in these patients. Patients with ZES have been treated continuously for up to 9 years with omeprazole with no loss of efficacy and no drug-related side-effects (Metz et al, 1993d (Figure 1). There is an extensive experience with the use of histamine H_2-receptor antagonists (cimetidine, ranitidine, famotidine) acquired prior to the introduction of the H^+–K^+-ATPase inhibitors (Jensen and Gardner, 1993; Metz and Jensen, 1995). Histamine H_2-receptor antagonists will control gastric acid hypersecretion in almost every patient with ZES; however, frequent (every 4–6 hours) high doses are almost always required (Jensen and Gardner, 1993; Metz et al, 1993c; Metz and Jensen, 1995). In studies at the NIH the mean daily cimetidine dose required was 3.6 g, for ranitidine 1.2 g, and for famotidine 0.25 g (Jensen and Gardner, 1993). Octreotide can also control acid hypersecretion in patients with ZES (Jensen and Gardner, 1993); however, it requires parenteral administration and therefore is less convenient than the use of H^+–K^+-ATPase inhibitors and is rarely used.

Various criteria have been proposed for adequate control of gastric acid hypersecretion in patients with ZES (Jensen and Gardner, 1993; Wolfe and Jensen, 1987; Raufman et al, 1983; Jensen et al, 1983b; Metz and Jensen, 1995; Metz et al, 1993). However, at present almost everyone uses the criterion of reduction of gastric acid secretion to less than 10 mEq/hour for the hour prior to the next dose of gastric antisecretory drug (Jensen et al, 1983b; Raufman et al, 1983; Wolfe and Jensen, 1987; Jensen and Gardner, 1993; Metz et al, 1993c; Metz and Jensen, 1995). In patients with severe reflux oesophagitis symptoms and/or disease, or who underwent a previous Billroth II procedure, gastric acid hypersecretion needs to be reduced to <5 mEq/hour and in some cases to <1 mEq/hour to control symptoms adequately (Maton et al, 1988; Miller et al, 1990; Jensen and Gardner, 1993; Metz and Jensen, 1995).

Some patients with ZES are acutely ill at presentation and parenteral gastric acid antisecretory therapy may be needed (London et al, 1989; Metz et al, 1993c). Parenteral omeprazole is highly effective (Vinayek et al, 1990, 1991) but is not presently available in the United States and therefore parenteral histamine H_2-receptor antagonists are routinely used in such a setting (Metz et al, 1993c; Metz and Jensen, 1995). Any of the histamine H_2-receptor antagonists can be used but the most extensive experience is with intravenous ranitidine (Vinayek et al, 1993) or cimetidine (Saeed et al, 1989). Usually a bolus injection of 150 mg of ranitidine is given, followed by a continuous intravenous infusion starting at 1 mg/kg body weight per hour (Vinayek et al, 1993). If cimetidine is used instead of ranitidine, a three fold higher dose is needed (Saeed et al, 1989). Acid secretion should be checked after several hours of starting the parenteral infusion and, if acid secretion is not controlled (<10 mEq/hour), the ranitidine dose should be increased at 0.5 mg/kg per hour increments. The mean dose of ranitidine is 1 mg/kg per hour with a range of 0.5–2.5 mg/kg per hour (Vinayek et al, 1993) and for cimetidine the mean dose was 1.9 mg/kg per hour with a range of 0.5–7.0 mg/kg per hour (Saeed et al, 1989). Patients with ZES have had acid secretion controlled for up to 2 months with parenteral histamine H_2-receptor antagonists using this approach, without side-effects (Saeed et al, 1989; Vinayek et al, 1993).

Post-curative resection of a gastrinoma by 3–6 months post-resection MAO decreased by 40% and BAO decreased by 75% (Pisegna et al, 1992). However, even with follow-up to 4 years post-resection, 67% of patients in one study (Pisegna et al, 1992) post-curative resection remained mild gastric acid hypersecretors (BAO <30 mEq/hour, mean 14 mEq/hour) and required low doses of ranitidine. The cause for this continued mild hyper-secretion or whether with longer follow-up it will disappear remain unclear (Pisegna et al, 1992).

Surgical management of acid hypersecretion

Total gastrectomy, which in the past was the standard treatment, should now be reserved for the rare patient who will not or cannot take regular oral medication (Bonfils et al, 1989; Jensen and Gardner, 1993). At present a total gastrectomy is relatively safe in a patient with ZES (Thompson et al, 1983). The operative mortality was 5.6% in 248 cases reported since 1980 and 2.4% for elective cases (Thompson et al, 1983). The morbidity is unclear but in some studies up to 50% have moderate to severe side-effects (Jensen and Gardner, 1993). Parietal cell vagotomy (PCV) at the time of the surgical exploration to remove the gastrinoma has been recommended (Richardson et al, 1985) and it was shown to result in a mean decrease in BAO of 41% and doses of antisecretory drugs could be reduced by 40%. However, in this initial study (Richardson et al, 1985) no patient was able to discontinue all antisecretory drugs (Richardson et al, 1985). With the subsequent availability of more potent histamine H_2-receptor antagonists and, more recently, H^+–K^+-ATPase inhibitors, PCV has been rarely used. A recent long-term follow-up of these patients (McArthur et al, 1996) demonstrates that 36% have been able to discontinue all antisecretory drugs; 86% of the patients continued to have reduced BAOs by 80% from the pre-operative level. This led the authors to propose that PCV should now be routinely used at the time of laparotomy. An accompanying editorial (Jensen, 1996) agreed with this conclusion, pointing out the value to the patients who were able to stop all drugs, importance of reduced drug expense, and avoidance of the need for long-term H^+–K^+-ATPase treatment with a successful PCV. This editorial (Jensen, 1996) also recommended PCV be considered in all patients undergoing curative resection.

Treatment of the gastrinoma

General

After control of the acid secretion is achieved, to treat the gastrinoma adequately in a patient with ZES, the tumour's location and the extent of the gastrinoma need to be established (Jensen and Gardner, 1993; Orbuch et al, 1995). Tumour extent assessment is essential to determine whether liver metastases are present, whether surgical resection of the primary tumour should be attempted, whether cytoreductive surgery for more extensive disease needs to be considered, or whether the tumour is extensive enough that tumoricidal treatment is required (Jensen and Gardner, 1993; Orbuch et al, 1995). Localization of the primary tumour is needed because these tumours are frequently small and multiple and can be difficult to find at laparotomy. Once tumour localization is accomplished, appropriate treatment of the gastrinoma needs to be undertaken because it may be possible to cure the patient by surgery (Norton et al, 1992; Jensen and Gardner, 1993; Fraker and Jensen, in press). Furthermore, surgical resection may extend life (Fraker et al, 1994) because these tumours are malignant in 60–90% of cases in older studies (Ellison and Wilson, 1964; Creutzfeldt et al, 1975; Jensen and Gardner, 1993), and recent studies show that the presence of liver metastases is related to the size of the primary tumour (Weber et al, 1995b). If extensive hepatic metastases are present, treatment directed against the tumour needs to be considered because the presence of liver metastases is the most important factor in determining prognosis (Weber et al, 1995b).

Tumour localization

Conventional imaging studies (bone scan, ultrasound, computerized tomography (CT) scan, magnetic resonance imaging (MRI), abdominal angiography) were the principal modalities used to localize the tumour pre-operatively until recently (Jensen and Gardner, 1993; Orbuch et al, 1995). Functional localization studies have also been used by measuring venous gastrin gradients either after percutaneous transhepatic sampling of the portal venous system (PVS) or after the intra-arterial injection (IAS) of secretin with hepatic venous sampling for gastrin levels. Functional localization methods have been used both to localize the primary tumour (Miller et al, 1992; Imamura and Takahashi, 1993; Strader et al, 1995) and to localize metastatic gastrinomas to the liver (Gibril et al, 1996). Recently two newer localization methods, endoscopic ultrasound (Ruszniewski et al, 1995a,b) and radionuclide scanning after intravenous injection of radio-labelled octreotide ([111In-DTPA-D-Phe1]octreotide) (somatostatin receptor scintigraphy (SRS)) (Krenning et al, 1993; de Kerviler et al, 1994;

Krenning et al, 1994; Gibril et al, in press), are increasingly used. More than 90% of gastrinomas have somatostatin receptors and SRS has been reported to be a particularly sensitive method to image gastrinomas, as well as most other PETs (Krenning et al, 1993; Ur et al, 1993; Krenning et al, 1994; Gibril et al, 1996a). It has been difficult to compare the sensitivities and specificities of SRS with the conventional imaging studies because in most studies only some procedures are done, the most sensitive conventional imaging studies such as angiography were rarely done, many studies have only small numbers of patients and the patients may vary in disease extent in different studies (Gibril et al, 1996a). Recently a large prospective NIH study (Gibril et al, 1996a) without these shortcomings evaluated the sensitivity of conventional imaging studies (ultrasound, CT scan, MRI, selective angiography) and SRS in 80 consecutive patients with ZES that allow a direct comparison of the different localization methods. These data are included in Table 3 with data from other studies. In analysing the results of imaging studies, it is important to consider the abilities of the different modalities to image the primary gastrinoma

Table 3. Ability of localization methods to identify gastrinomas in patients with Zollinger–Ellison syndrome.

| | Sensitivity (%)[a] | | |
| | | Literature | |
Localization modality	1996 NIH SRS Study[b]	Mean	(Range)
I. Extrahepatic lesion identified			
Ultrasound	9*	23	(21–28)
CT scan	31*	38	(0–59)
MRI	30*	22	(20–25)
Angiography	28*	68	(35–68)
SRS	58	72	(58–77)
Endoscopic ultrasound	—	70	(16–86)
Intra-arterial secretin test	—	89	(55–100)
PVS	—	68	(60–94)
Intra-operative ultrasound	—	83	(75–100)
II. Metastatic liver disease identified			
Ultrasound	46*	14	(14–63)
CT scan	42*	54	(35–72)
MRI	71	63	(43–83)
Angiography	65*	62	(33–86)
SRS	92	97	(92–100)
IAS	—	40	

* <0.05 compared with SRS alone.
SRS data from de Kervilar et al (1994), Krenning et al (1994) and Gibril et al (1996a). Endoscopic ultrasound from Thompson et al, (1994), de Kervilar et al (1994) and Ruszniewski et al (1995a). IAS for liver metastases from Gibril et al (1996b). Other imaging studies from Norton et al (1986a), Frucht et al (1990), Miller et al (1992), Jenson and Gardner (1993), Sugg et al (1993), Krenning et al (1994), Norton (1995), Orbuch et al (1995) and Strader et al (1995).
[a] Sensitivity is expressed as the percentage of patients with positive tumour localization with the indicated modality.
[b] Data from the NIH study comparing the ability of SRS with CT, MRI, ultrasound and selective angiography to localize an extrahepatic gastrinoma or the presence of proven liver metastases in 80 consecutive patients with ZES (Gibril et al, 1996a).

separately from their ability to localize gastrinoma metastatic to the liver (Jensen and Gardner, 1993; Gibril et al, 1996a). Metastatic liver lesions are frequently imaged to determine the need for treatment directed against the tumour, to determine that exploratory laparotomy for cure is not indicated, and to assess the results of anti-tumour therapy, whereas primary tumours are imaged to determine potential resectability.

In the recent NIH study of 80 consecutive cases (Gibril et al, 1996a), ultrasound, CT scan, MRI and angiography localized an extrahepatic lesion in less than 50% of cases (Table 3); however, similarly to previous studies using these modalities, their specificities were high (Jensen and Gardner, 1993; Orbuch et al, 1995). The SRS has greater sensitivity than any single conventional imaging study (Table 3) and in the recent NIH study (Gibril et al, 1996a) it was equal in sensitivity for localizing an extrahepatic gastrinoma to all the conventional imaging studies combined. Figure 4 shows the results of SRS in a patient with negative conventional imaging studies in which the SRS localized a gastrinoma in the pancreatic head area, and subsequently at surgery a gastrinoma was found in a lymph node in the pancreatic head area. Endoscopic ultrasound is reported to be particularly useful for identifying pancreatic gastrinomas (Thompson et al, 1994; Ruszniewski et al, 1995a) (Table 3). In a recent comparative study (de Kerviler et al, 1994) of 32 patients with ZES, SRS detected a pancreatico-duodenal gastrinoma in 56%, endoscopic ultrasound in 40%, and both together in 69%. In a recent study endoscopic ultrasound detected 50% of duodenal gastrinomas, 75% of the pancreatic tumours and 62% of the gastrinomas in lymph nodes (Ruszniewski et al, 1995a). Figure 5 demonstrates the results of endoscopic ultrasound in a patient with ZES in which conventional imaging studies were negative but SRS had showed a lesion in the pancreatic head–duodenal area. Endoscopic ultrasound demonstrated a periduodenal tumour in the same area as the SRS (Figure 5) and at surgery a gastrinoma was found in this area in a lymph node.

The ability of conventional imaging studies (ultrasound, CT scan, MRI, angiography) to identify any PET or gastrinoma is dependent on tumour size (Orbuch et al, 1995). With tumours < 1 cm in diameter no tumours are generally seen, with a tumour diameter of 1–3 cm 15–30% are seen, and with tumours > 3 cm in diameter 95–100% are detected (Orbuch et al, 1995). Therefore, conventional imaging studies miss most duodenal gastrinomas which are characteristically <1 cm (Thom et al, 1991; Weber et al, 1995b). In two studies CT scan detected only 9% of duodenal tumours in one study (Ruszniewski et al, 1995a) and in another study (Sugg et al, 1993) of 35 patients with surgically proven duodenal gastrinomas, the combination of ultrasound, CT scan and MRI identified a tumour in only 15% of the patients, and selective angiography in 47% of the patients. In many cases it is likely that the angiogram was actually identifying tumour in lymph nodes which occurred in 60% of the patients, not the small duodenal tumour. Recent studies (Thompson et al, 1994; Ruszniewski et al, 1995a) suggest that both endoscopic ultrasound and SRS may also miss more than 50% of all duodenal gastrinomas.

In contrast to conventional imaging studies, functional localization

CT

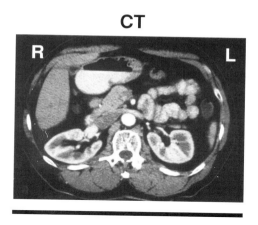

SRS

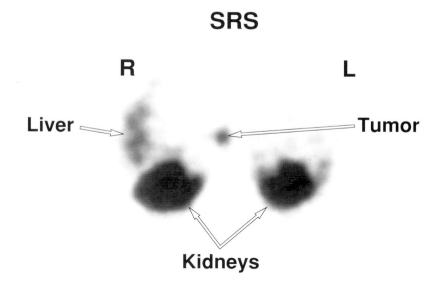

Figure 4. Ability of CT scan and SRS to localize a gastrinoma in a patient with ZES. The CT scan (top panel) demonstrated no gastrinoma in this patient (NIH 2815104), whereas a tumour is identified on the SRS in the lower panel. At surgery a 2 cm gastrinoma was found in a pancreatic head lymph node and the patient has remained cured post-operatively.

studies are not dependent on tumour size (Strader et al, 1995). Hepatic venous sampling after selective intra-arterial injection of secretin was more frequently positive for localizing an extrahepatic tumor than PVS (89% versus 68%) (Table 3). With duodenal gastrinomas, compared with PVS,

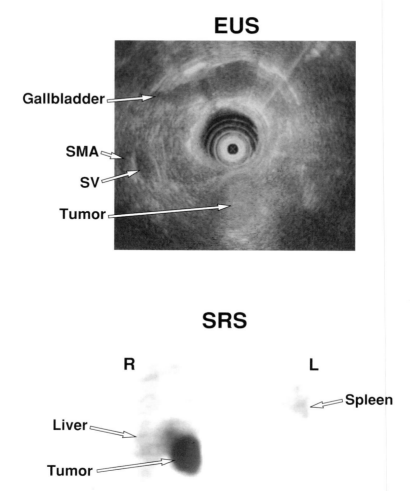

Figure 5. Ability of endoscopic ultrasound (EUS) and SRS to localize a gastrinoma in a patient with ZES. Endoscopic ultrasound (top panel) demonstrated a 2 cm pancreatic head tumour probably in a lymph node (labelled 'tumour'). In the bottom panel in the same area, SRS demonstrates a tumour. In this patient (NIH 2946750) at surgery a 2.5 cm pancreatic head lymph node positive for gastrinoma was removed in the same area indicated by the EUS and the SRS and also a small duodenal gastrinoma was removed which was not seen by either modality. The patient was cured at post-operative evaluation.

the intra-arterial secretin test was more frequently positive (78% versus 28%) (Thom et al, 1992). Similarly, in a recent study (Sugg et al, 1993) on localizing duodenal gastrinomas, the intra-arterial secretin test was the most sensitive localization method (96%), having greater sensitivity than PVS (77%) and conventional imaging studies (52%). It has been recently proposed that because of its increased sensitivity, ease of performance and lower complication rate, the intra-arterial secretin should replace PVS in patients with ZES (Thom et al, 1992; Strader et al, 1995). Functional localization for hepatic metastases has also been reported using injections of secretin into the hepatic arteries (Gibril et al, 1996b). In a recent study (Gibril et al, 1996b), criteria were developed for a positive gradient in such a study and although it had a lower sensitivity (41%) than CT (64%), ultrasound (64%), MRI (77%) or angiography (77%), the intra-arterial secretin test assisted in management in 22% of the patients. SRS was not assessed in this study (Gibril et al, 1996b). At present, functional localization studies are not routinely recommended (Strader et al, 1995) and it remains unclear whether they offer advantages over SRS. In the case of extrahepatic lesions, functional studies localize only to the general area and not to specific structures within this area (i.e. pancreatic area, not duodenum). Because >70% of gastrinomas are in the pancreatic head area, the study is primarily of assistance in the 30% outside this area. A functional study will probably continue to be particularly useful in two clinical situations. First, if a patient has MEN 1 and multiple tumours, functional localization will assist in excluding the 20% of gastrinomas outside the duodenum. Second, if a proximal pancreaticoduodenectomy (Whipple) is planned if no tumour is found at laparotomy, then functional studies establish the presence of gastrinoma only in this area (Strader et al, 1995).

For localizing metastatic disease in the liver, the recent NIH study (Gibril et al, 1996a) confirms the results of a number of previous studies (Krenning et al, 1993, 1994) demonstrating that SRS is the single most sensitive modality (Table 3). From these studies it can be concluded that SRS will identify >90% of patients with ZES with hepatic metastases (Table 3). In the recent NIH study (Gibril et al, 1996a) SRS was equal in sensitivity to the combination of all conventional studies for identifying patients with metastatic liver lesions (92% versus 83%). The sensitivity seen in the NIH study (Gibril et al, 1996a) with SRS can only be obtained if single photon emission computed tomographic scanning imaging is performed (Corleto et al, 1996). Recent improvements in MRI scanning have greatly increased its sensitivity for localizing hepatic metastases in patients with ZES. (Frucht et al, 1989a; Pisegna et al, 1993a). The use particularly of short inversion-time inversion recovery (STIR) sequences allows liver metastases to be easily seen (Pisegna et al, 1993a). A recent NIH study compared SRS with other imaging studies (Table 3) (Gibril et al, 1996a) and the SRS and MRI had similar sensitivities (92% versus 71%, $P = 0.12$). Therefore, if SRS is not available MR imaging should be done. An example of the use of SRS and MRI to image liver metastases is shown in Figure 6. This patient had a single right lobe liver metastasis which is well seen by both studies.

At exploratory laparotomy, three intra-operative procedures are currently used to assist in localizing gastrinomas. Intra-operative ultrasound (IOUS) is particularly helpful for identifying pancreatic gastrinomas, localizing 91% of pancreatic gastrinomas but only 30% of duodenal gastrinomas (Norton et al, 1988; Norton 1995). The use of IOUS altered surgical management in 10% of cases (Norton et al, 1988). In one prospective study at the NIH, transillumination of the duodenum at surgery allows duodenal

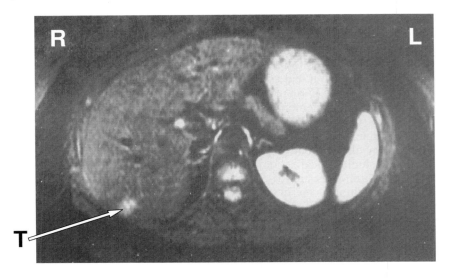

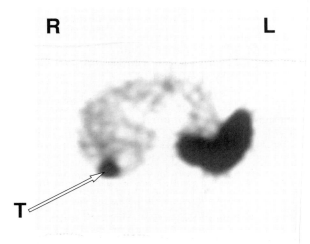

Figure 6. Ability of MRI and SRS to localize a liver metastasis in a patient with ZES. The top panel shows an MRI STIR image and the bottom panel shows the SRS result. A single right lobe liver metastasis is seen in both images (NIH 1923492). The MRI identified 71% and SRS 92% of patients with proven metastatic liver disease in a recent large study (Gibril et al, 1996a).

tumours to be localized (Frucht et al, 1990). In recent data from the NIH (Figure 7), transillumination of the duodenum at the time of surgery will detect 15% more duodenal gastrinomas than palpation alone (Frucht et al, 1990; Sugg et al, 1993) (Figure 7). Duodenotomy identifies 100% of all duodenal tumours and in our most recent data it localizes 25% more duodenal gastrinomas than palpation, IOUS and transillumination combined (Figure 7). It is now recommended that IOUS, duodenal transillumination and duodenotomy should be used in all ZES cases during surgical exploration (Norton 1994, 1995). Although duodenotomy will localize the duodenal tumours found by transillumination, the transillumination is still recommended because it guides placement of the duodenotomy site (Sugg et al, 1993).

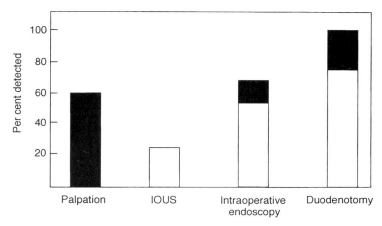

Figure 7. Intra-operative detection of duodenal gastrinomas. The ability of palpation (performed first), followed by IOUS, followed by intra-operative endoscopy with transillumination (intra-operative endoscopy) and duodenectomy to find a duodenal tumour in 75 consecutive patients with ZES was studied. Gastrinomas were found in 97% of the patients of which 48 patients had duodenal tumours. Results are expressed as the percentage of the duodenal tumours found by the indicated method, with the black portion representing the percentage of new tumours found by the indicated method and the white area representing the percentage localized by the indicated method that had been found with the previous methods. Palpation found 60% of the duodenal tumours, and 0% additional were found by IOUS, 15% by intra-operative endoscopy, and 25% by duodenotomy (data from the NIH, May 1996).

Treatment of the gastrinoma in patients with ZES without liver metastases with MEN 1

At present there is no agreement on the best method to treat the gastrinoma in patients with MEN 1 with ZES (Jensen and Gardner, 1993; Norton et al, 1993; Jensen, 1994; Metz et al, 1994). Until recently it was recommended that these patients not undergo routine exploratory laparotomy because they were rarely cured by tumour enucleation (Deveney et al, 1983; Jensen et al, 1983b; Malagelada et al, 1983; Jensen and Gardner, 1993; Norton et al, 1993; Jensen, 1994; Metz et al, 1994). A surgical approach to these patients was reconsidered in 1990 (Pipeleers-Marichal et al, 1990) when eight patients with ZES and MEN 1 were described, all of whom had only duodenal gastrinomas and post-resection normalized serum gastrin in four of the six patients. Pipeleers-Marichal et al (1990) proposed that patients with ZES with MEN 1 should have surgical explorations to remove the duodenal tumours. While this study called attention to the frequent occurrence of the gastrinoma in the duodenum in patients with MEN 1, its conclusions were limited by the short follow-up time and failure to perform secretin tests post-resection in all patients, which are needed to be certain that the patients are cured (Fishbeyn et al, 1993). Three recent studies provide additional data on this approach. In two studies (Ruszniewski et al, 1993b; MacFarlane et al, 1995; Mignon et al, 1995a) pancreatic gastrinomas were reported in 20% and 62% of patients with MEN 1 and ZES; therefore gastrinomas do not exclusively occur in the duodenum in patients with ZES with MEN 1. In a recent prospective study (MacFarlane et al, 1995) the ability to cure patients with MEN 1 and ZES surgically by careful duodenal exploration was assessed in 10 consecutive patients. All patients had gastrinomas found at exploration and 70% of patients had a duodenal gastrinoma, 20% a pancreatic gastrinoma, and 10% a gastrinoma only in lymph nodes. No patient was cured post-resection. Failure to cure these patients occurred because 86% of the duodenal gastrinomas had metastasized to lymph nodes, 30% of patients had >20 duodenal gastrinomas and enucleation of the pancreatic gastrinomas did not result in cure, suggesting there must be either retained metastases to lymph nodes or multiple primaries (MacFarlane et al, 1995). This study (MacFarlane et al, 1995) clearly demonstrates that patients with ZES with MEN 1 cannot be cured by gastrinoma enucleation alone. Some groups (Delcore and Friesen, 1994; Stadil, 1995) recommend that a Whipple resection should be considered in patients with ZES with MEN 1 and in one study (Stadil, 1995) three such patients remained cured for 7, 9 and 13 years post-resection. At present this recommendation is not generally endorsed (Norton and Jensen, 1991; Jensen and Gardner, 1993; Jensen, 1994). The principal difficulty in generally endorsing this procedure is that it remains unclear what the natural histories of the PETs are in patients with MEN 1. Therefore, it remains unclear whether any surgical intervention prolongs survival. In the case of ZES in a patient with MEN 1 in which the symptoms of acid hypersecretion can be controlled effectively by oral anti-secretory medications, the question of whether resection of the gastrinoma alone reduces the rate of metastatic disease and prolongs life remains un-answered.

Treatment of the gastrinoma in patients with ZES without liver metastases or MEN 1

Until recently, the role of routine surgical exploration in patients with ZES without MEN 1 or medical contraindications to surgery was controversial but in contrast to the situation with patients with MEN 1 with ZES, recent studies have provided clarification (McCarthy, 1980; Norton and Jensen, 1991; Jensen and Gardner, 1993; Jensen, 1994; Hirschowitz, 1995). Controversy existed in large part, primarily because of three different un-resolved areas (Fishbeyn et al, 1993; Jensen and Gardner, 1993; Fraker et al, 1994; Hirschowitz, 1995). First, there was an uncertainty about long-term cure rates post-resection in patients without MEN 1 (Fishbeyn et al,

1993; Jensen and Gardner, 1993; Fraker et al, 1994; Hirschowitz, 1995). Second, there was a failure of any surgical studies to demonstrate for patients with ZES or any malignant PET that early surgical removal of the primary tumour decreased the development of metastases or extended survival. Third, there was a lack of agreement on the natural history of gastrinomas in these patients. Within the last few years studies have provided partial answers to each of these questions and support the recommendation that all patients with ZES without metastatic liver disease, MEN 1 or medical contraindications to surgery or limiting life expectancy should undergo surgical exploration for possible cure (Wolfe and Jensen, 1987; Jensen and Gardner, 1993; Jensen and Fraker, 1994; Norton 1994). First, at least three studies Fraker et al, 1994; Weber et al, 1995b; McArthur et al, 1996) now provide long-term follow-up data on patients with ZES after undergoing surgical explorations ($N = 120$) or not ($N = 28$). The data from a large NIH study (Weber et al, 1995b) are particularly helpful because they demonstrates that in 75% of patients the gastrinoma pursues a relatively non-aggressive course, whereas in 25% it follows an aggressive course. In this study (Weber et al, 1995b) the aggressive form was found to occur more frequently in females, to be uncommon in patients with MEN 1, to be associated with a short onset time to diagnosis, and to be associated with much higher serum gastrin elevations, larger tumours (>3 cm diameter) and tumours that were pancreatic in location. The 10-year survival was 30% in the aggressive form compared with 96% in patients with the non-aggressive form of the disease. The presence of lymph node metastases did not distinguish the non-aggressive and aggressive forms, only the presence of liver metastases. Another study (Metz et al, 1993a) demonstrated that the aggressive form is associated with certain flow cytometry results including a high S phase, low percentage non-tetraploid aneuploid and a higher percentage of multiple stem line aneuploid. Despite these differences between the non-aggressive and aggressive forms of ZES, it is not possible to predict in an individual patient what course the disease will take. Second, a recent NIH study provides evidence for the first time that surgical excision decreases the rate of development of metastases in patients with ZES (Fraker et al, 1994). In this study only 3/98 patients (3%) undergoing surgery for cure developed liver metastases, whereas 6/26 patients (23%) ($P < 0.0003$) not undergoing surgery developed hepatic metastases (Figure 8). Furthermore, patients undergoing resection had almost ($P = 0.085$) significantly longer survival than patients without surgery ($P = 0.085$) (Fraker et al, 1994) (Figure 8). This study was not a randomized study; however, the two groups were well matched for clinical characteristics, time of onset to follow-up (15.4 versus 14.0 years) and time since diagnosis (9.4 versus 7.7 years). The percentage of patients with MEN 1 in the no-operation group was numerically higher, but the difference was not significant (35% versus 15%, $P > 0.05$). Lastly, data now exist on short- and long-term surgical cure rates. At present gastrinomas are found at surgery in >90% of cases, and, in the most recent NIH study, 60% of patients were disease free immediately post-operatively and 30% at five years (Norton et al, 1992; Fishbeyn et al, 1993). These results can only be obtained if a thorough search of the duodenum is performed including the routine use of duodenotomy (Sugg et al, 1993; Jensen and Fraker, 1994) (Figure 7). In a recent study (Jensen and Fraker, 1994) of 42 patients with ZES of which gastrinomas were found in 95%, 71% of the patients had duodenal tumours. In our last 75 patients undergoing exploratory laparotomy, of which 97% had a gastrinoma found, 64% had a duodenal tumour (Figure 7). Palpation alone found 60% of the duodenal tumours, IOUS localized no new duodenal tumours, endoscopic transillumination an additional 15%, and duodenotomy an additional 25% (Figure 7). These results demonstrate that routine duodenotomy should now be performed in all patients with ZES undergoing exploratory laparotomy.

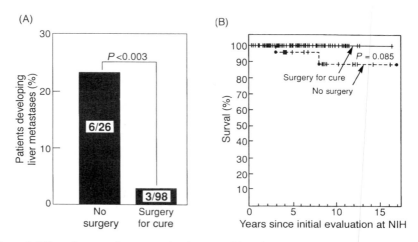

Figure 8. Effect of surgery for cure on development of hepatic metastases and survival in patients with ZES. (A) Percentage of patients medically managed without surgical exploration for cure ($N = 26$), and percentage of patients undergoing surgery for cure ($N = 98$) who developed hepatic metastases during follow-up (mean 7 years). (B) Survival in these two groups of patients. Data from Fraker et al (1994).

Treatment of the gastrinoma in patients with ZES with liver metastases

General. Similarly to other malignant PETs, gastrinomas are usually considered a slow-growing tumour; however, in recent studies the five-year survival of patients with metastatic liver disease is as low as 20% (Jensen and Gardner, 1993; Norton et al, 1993). With the increased ability to control acid secretion, the natural history of the gastrinoma now is increasingly becoming the primary determinant of survival (Jensen and Gardner, 1993; Norton et al, 1993). There is thus an increasing need for effective treatment of metastatic disease. Numerous treatments have been recommended including chemotherapy, systematic removal of all resectable tumour (cytoreductive surgery), treatment with the long-acting somatostatin analogue, octreotide, treatment with interferon, hepatic embolization alone or with chemotherapy (chemoembolization), and liver transplantation

(Jensen and Gardner, 1993; Oberg, 1993; Arcenas et al, 1995; Arnold and Frank, 1995; Azoulay and Bismuth, 1995; Jensen, 1995; Nagorney and Que, 1995; Fraker and Jensen, in press). Treatment with each of these modalities has been reviewed recently (Fraker and Jensen, in press) including with chemotherapy (Arnold and Frank, 1995), cytoreductive surgery (Nagorney and Que, 1995), vascular occlusion (Arcenas et al, 1995), liver transplantation (Azoulay and Bismuth, 1995), treatment with octreotide (Arnold et al, 1992, 1993), and interferon (Eriksson and Oberg, 1995) and thus will be discussed only briefly below. At the current time the role of each of these modalities in the treatment of patients with metastatic gastrinoma remains unclear (Jensen and Gardner, 1993; Norton et al, 1993; Fraker and Jensen, in press). Although different treatments have been compared with each other and superiority shown, because of the variable course of different patients it still remains unclear how much advantage a given treatment has over no treatment.

Chemotherapy. With different types of PETs, including gastrinomas, except with streptozotocin and chlorozotocin, single-agent chemotherapy has had low success rates (Norton et al, 1993; Oberg 1993; Fraker and Jensen, in press). Streptozotocin (Moertel et al, 1980; Jensen et al, 1983b) and chlorozotocin (Moertel et al, 1992) alone have given response rates of 25–50%. Combinations of streptozotocin or chlorozotocin in patients with a variety of PETs have been evaluated in a number of studies (Bukowski et al, 1992; Norton et al, 1993; Oberg, 1993; Arnold and Frank, 1995; Fraker and Jensen, in press). In a prospective Eastern Cooperative Oncology Group (ECOG) study (Moertel et al, 1980) the combination of streptozotocin plus 5-fluorouracil gave a better response rate than streptozotocin alone (63% versus 40% response rate). A subsequent ECOG study (Moertel et al, 1992) in patients with a variety of malignant PETs demonstrated that streptozotocin plus doxorubicin was superior to streptozotocin plus 5-fluorouracil or chlorozotocin alone (response rates of 69%, 45% and 30%, respectively). The median durations of tumour regression were 18 months, 14 months, and 17 months, respectively; however, the survival time for patients treated with the doxorubicin combination was longer (Moertel et al, 1992). Streptozotocin plus 5-fluorouracil (Broder and Carter, 1973; Hofmann et al, 1973; Mignon et al, 1986; Ruszniewski et al, 1991), streptozotocin plus doxorubicin (Moertel et al, 1992), and streptozotocin plus both drugs (von Schrenck et al, 1988) have been used in small numbers of patients with metastatic gastrinomas in various series with response rates varying from 5% to 80% (Norton et al, 1993; Fraker and Jensen, in press). However, in two prospective studies involving only patients with metastatic gastrinoma (Bonfils et al, 1986; von Schrenck et al, 1988), the response rates were 5% and 40%, which are lower than reported in the ECOG studies which involved patients with a number of different malignant PETs. The combination of etoposide and cisplatin (Moertel et al, 1991) is reported to give a response rate in 67% of anaplastic neuroendocrine tumours; however, the response rate in metastatic gastrinomas was 16% (Moertel et al, 1991).

Hepatic embolization with or without chemotherapy. Hepatic embolization with or without chemotherapy has been reported to be of value in a small number of patients with metastatic gastrinomas and other PETs (Carrasco et al, 1983; Norton et al, 1993; Perry et al, 1994; Arcenas et al, 1995; Fraker and Jensen, in press). Because the liver derives only 20–25% of its blood supply from the hepatic artery and 75–80% from the portal vein and because most PETs including gastrinomas are vascular with an arterial supply, hepatic artery embolization can be used if the portal vein is patent. In combined series of PETs, 68–100% of patients are reported to show improvement with this treatment (Moertel et al, 1994; Fraker and Jensen, in press). Recently chemoembolization with doxorubicin in iodized oil combined with either sponge particles or gelatin powder has been reported to decrease tumour size in 57–100% of patients (Carrasco et al, 1983; Stokes et al, 1993; Perry et al, 1994; Fraker and Jensen, in press). In a recent study (Ruszniewski et al, 1993b) five patients with metastatic gastrinoma in the liver were treated with such a regimen. In contrast to patients with carcinoid tumours ($N = 18$) in which symptoms of the carcinoid syndrome were controlled by such treatment in 80% and size of liver metastases decreased by 50% in one-half of the patients, in patients with ZES 60% (three of five patients) had a minor response ($N = 1$) or stabilization ($N = 2$). The authors of this study (Ruszniewski et al, 1993b) concluded that gastrinomas may be less responsive to chemoembolization than carcinoid tumours, although the experience was limited.

Cytoreductive surgery. Removal of all resectable tumour has long been recommended for treating metastatic PETs (McEntee et al, 1990; Carty et al, 1992; Nagorney and Que, 1995; Que et al, 1995). A number of recent studies (Norton et al, 1986b; McEntee et al, 1990; Carty et al, 1992; Que et al, 1995) and a recent review (Nagorney and Que, 1995) have provided support for such an approach. In one study (Carty et al, 1992) involving 17 cases with potentially resectable PETs, in 80% of the cases the tumour was completely resected and survival was 79% at five years. Unfortunately only a small proportion of all patients with PETs fall into the potentially resectable category (i.e. 9% in one study (McEntee et al, 1990) and 5% in another (Carty et al, 1992)). This approach has been advocated in patients with ZES with potentially resectable metastatic liver disease (Zollinger et al, 1980; Norton et al, 1986b). In one study (Norton et al, 1986b) 20% of patients with metastatic liver disease with ZES were potentially resectable on tumour imaging studies; each patient underwent hepatic resection and two patients maintained normal serum gastrin levels post-resection. These data, as well as experience with other PETs, suggest that, if imaging studies determine that the metastatic disease is confined to one liver lobe and the primary tumour is resectable, or if more than 90% of the imaged tumour can be safely resected, surgical resection should be attempted.

Treatment with interferon. Interferon is effective at both controlling symptoms and also inhibiting further tumour growth of metastatic PETs in a number of studies (Eriksson et al, 1986; Norton et al, 1993; Pisegna et al,

1993b; Eriksson and Oberg, 1995; Fraker and Jensen, in press). In a recent review (Eriksson and Oberg, 1995) of a number of series involving 322 patients with various neuroendocrine tumours, 43% showed a biochemical response (<50% decrease in hormone levels), and 12% showed a decrease in tumour size with interferon. Interferon has been used in a small number of patients with metastatic gastrinoma (Eriksson et al, 1986; Pisegna et al, 1993b). In one recent pre-operative study (Pisegna et al, 1993b) of 11 patients with metastatic gastrinoma increasing in size in the liver, with treatment with daily α-interferon (5 million units/day) no patient had a decrease in tumour size, but three patients (30%) had a stabilization of tumour size. These results and those in other metastatic PETs demonstrate that interferon rarely causes a decrease in tumour size, but probably has a tumoristatic effect in some patients resulting in stabilization of the metastatic disease in 25–30%. Whether interferon treatment results in prolonged survival is not established.

Treatment with somatostatin analogues. More than 90% of gastrinomas as well as other PETs, except insulinomas, possess somatostatin receptors (Bruns et al, 1994; Krenning et al, 1994; Reubi et al, 1994; Scarpignato, 1995; Lamberts et al, 1996; Fraker and Jensen, in press) which mediate the action of somatostatin on these tumours. Two long-acting somatostatin analogues have been used in clinical studies, lanreotide and octreotide (Anthony et al, 1993; Lamberts et al, 1996). Recent studies provide evidence for five somatostatin receptor subtypes and the actions of these two long-acting somatostatin analogues are primarily mediated by subtype 2 (Bruns et al, 1994; Reubi et al, 1994; Lamberts et al, 1996). In a recent review of 66 patients treated with octreotide with metastatic neuro-endocrine tumours, octreotide caused a decrease in tumour size in 12% of patients (eight patients); however, in other studies it caused a disease stabilization in 25–50% (Kvols et al, 1987; Maton, 1989; Maton et al, 1989a; Arnold et al, 1993; Saltz et al, 1993; Arnold et al, 1994; Fraker and Jensen, in press). Similar studies have been performed on a small number of patients with metastatic gastrinoma (Arnold et al, 1993; Saltz et al, 1993; Arnold et al, 1994; Fraker and Jensen, in press). One recent study (Arnold et al, 1996) involving 65 patients with metastatic liver disease due to a malignant neuroendocrine tumour (52 patients with progressive disease, 13 patients with stable disease), octreotide caused disease stabilization in 36% of those with progressive disease for at least 3 months. These data suggest that long-acting somatostatin analogues probably have a tumoristatic effect in some patients with metastatic gastrinoma, however rarely have a tumoricidal effect resulting in a decreasing tumour size. Whether treatment with somatostatin analogues prolongs life is not established.

Liver transplantation. Liver transplantation has been reported in a small number of patients with metastatic PETs and with metastatic gastrinomas (Azoulay and Bismuth, 1995; Dousset et al, 1995; Jensen, 1995; Routley et al, 1995). Each of these reports has only a small number of cases (<11 patients). Most reports recommend that liver transplantation be considered in selected doses, particularly patients without extrahepatic disease. It appears from the small number of cases ($N = 23$) that long-term cure is uncommon, with recurrence to bone, lymph nodes or liver most common. However, in a recent (Anthuber et al, 1996) study involving four patients with metastatic PETs (no gastrinomas) undergoing transplantation, no patient survived beyond 33 months. Three died from tumour recurrence and one died of a fungal infection and at autopsy had spine metastases that had been missed. The authors conclude that their results do not support the promising data of others and recommend that liver transplantation in these patients should only be done in carefully selected patients. Therefore, at present it remains unclear which patients, if any, with metastatic gastrinoma or other PETs should undergo liver transplantation. It may be possible with the recent availability of SRS better to select patients who do not have distant metastases that would be missed in the past with less sensitive imaging methods.

RECENT ADVANCES

General

Recent advances in areas related to the diagnosis, clinical presentation, differential diagnosis and aspects of treatment (including tumour localization, treatment of the gastric acid hypersecretion, surgical treatment of gastrinomas, treatment of ZES with MEN 1, and treatment for metastatic disease) were integrated into these specific sections in the paper.

One area not dealt with in these sections, where recent important insights are occurring, is the area of gastrinoma cell biology as well as that of other related PETs, and this will be briefly covered in the next section.

Tumour biology of gastrinoma and other PETs

Gastrinomas resemble other PETs and carcinoid tumours in being neuroendocrine neoplasms which share certain features (Norton et al, 1993; Kloppel et al, 1995). All of these tumours can be classified as APUDomas (amine precursor uptake and decarboxylation) because they share the expression of genes encoding certain markers and hormonal products such as chromogranin A and B, synaptophysin, neuron-specific enolase, 7B2 and epitole Leu-7 (Kloppel et al, 1995). Their malignancy potential cannot be predicted from histological, ultrastructural or immunocytochemical studies (Jensen and Gardner, 1993; Jensen and Norton, 1995; Kloppel et al, 1995). The only reliable criterion of malignancy is the presence of metastases.

The cell of origin of gastrinomas, as well as these other PETs, remains unclear. Recent studies suggest that duodenal and pancreatic gastrinomas, which differ in biological behaviour (Jensen and Gardner, 1993; Weber et al, 1995b) may also differ in their cells of origin. A recent study (Howard et al, 1995) provides evidence that duodenal gastrinomas probably arise from the pancreatic ventral bud tissue and pancreatic gastrinomas arise from the dorsal pancreatic bud tissue.

Gastrinomas, like other PETs, frequently release additional peptides into the circulation as well as gastrin, with 62% of all patients with ZES in one study (Chiang et al, 1990) releasing at least one additional hormone and 100% of untreated patients releasing chromogranin A (Syversen et al, 1993; Eriksson, 1995). The additional release of peptides occasionally causes a second hormone syndrome but in patients without MEN 1, except for ectopic Cushing's syndrome in patients with advanced disease, a second hormonal syndrome is uncommon (Maton et al, 1986; Chiang et al, 1990).

Because of the inability to determine malignancy without establishing the presence of metastases, numerous attempts to predict malignant behaviour from tumour markers, analysis of gastrin-like peptides or precursors and molecular studies are being increasingly investigated. α and β subunits of human chorionic gonadotropin (α-HCG, β-HCG) are elevated in 41% and 30% of patients with ZES and their presence correlates with malignancy in one study (Eriksson, 1995), but not in another (Jensen and Gardner, 1993). Higher plasma progastrin levels (Bardram, 1990a; Jensen and Gardner, 1993), lower percentage amidated gastrin (Bardram, 1990a; Jensen and Gardner, 1993) and the NH_2:COOH terminal gastrin ratio (Bardram, 1990b; Jensen and Gardner, 1993) have all been proposed to be predictive of malignancy; however, there is so much variability in a given case that a single determination has little diagnostic value (Bardram, 1990b; Jensen and Gardner, 1993; Rehfeld and Bardram, 1995). A recent clinical study (Weber et al, 1995b) provides important insights into the effect of gastrinoma location or size on malignancy potential. This study (Weber et al, 1995b) demonstrated that the presence of liver metastases was highly dependent on the primary tumour size ($P < 0.000\,01$) and location ($P < 0.000\,01$). Pancreatic, but not duodenal, gastrinomas are frequently large (>3 cm) and are associated frequently with hepatic metastases (Weber et al, 1995b). Interestingly, the percentage of duodenal and pancreatic gastrinomas with lymph node metastases did not vary (i.e. 48% versus 47%). Furthermore, this study (Weber et al, 1995b) demonstrated that in 25% of patients the ZES pursues an aggressive course and in 75% a non-aggressive course. Patients with tumours having an aggressive course developed liver metastases and had a 10-year survival of 30% (Weber et al, 1995b). The presence or absence of lymph node metastases had no effect on survival.

Gastrinoma cells are difficult to grow in culture so there are no data on the direct effect of growth factors on tumour growth. Various recent studies show that gastrinomas, similarly to other PETs, make growth factors such as PDGE, $TGF\beta_1$, β_2 β_2 and bFGF, as well as possessing growth factor receptors (Oberg 1994; Chaudhry and Oberg, 1995). In addition, all gastrinomas in one study (Chaudhry et al, 1994) express the hyaluronate receptor CD44 (Chaudhry et al, 1994; Chaudhry and Oberg, 1995) which in some tumours correlated with the tendency to metastasize to lymph nodes (Chaudhry et al, 1994). Furthermore, gastrinomas more frequently overproduced a larger molecular weight splice variant of CD44 than other PETs (Chaudhry et al, 1994).

Recent studies demonstrate that various tumour suppressor genes and proto-oncogenes may play a role in the pathogenesis of some endocrine tumours (Arnold, 1994; Evers et al, 1994; Weber and Jensen, 1996). Recently the proto-oncogene *HER-2/neu*, which is a member of the *erb*-β-like oncogene family that encodes a protein (p185[neu]) with tyrosine kinase activity, was examined in 11 gastrinomas (Evers et al, 1994). It was over-expressed (>2-fold) in all gastrinomas; however, the overexpression did not correlate with aggressiveness as has been shown in some breast cancers. In contrast, no alteration in *K-ras*, *N-ras*, *H-ras* was shown in 23 gastrinomas in two studies (Yashiro et al, 1993; Evers et al, 1994) and only rarely have p53 mutations been found in gastrinomas as well as other PETs (Weber and Jensen, 1996). Recently, alterations in the expression of guanine nucleotide binding proteins ($G\alpha_s$, $G\alpha_{i2}$) have been reported in a number of endocrine tumours (Landis et al, 1989; Lyons et al, 1990; Vessey et al, 1994). However, no alterations in either G protein were found in two gastrinomas or nine insulinomas in a recent study (Vessey et al, 1994). However, the mRNA of the α subunit of G_s was overexpressed (Zeiger and Norton, 1993) in an ACTHoma and an insulinoma but not a gastrinoma in one study. Lastly, recent studies provide evidence that loss of heterozygosity on chromosome 11q12–13 near the PYGM locus may be important in the pathogenesis of both sporadic gastrinomas and other sporadic PETs as it is in the case of patients with MEN 1 (Sawicki et al, 1992; Bale, 1994; Eubanks et al, 1994; Weber and Jensen, 1996). In one study (Sawicki et al, 1992), five of 11 sporadic gastrinomas had a loss of heterozygosity in this area, and in another study (Eubanks et al, 1994) 30% of sporadic PETs had a loss of heterozygosity in the region of the putative MEN 1 gene.

SUMMARY

Since the description of the Zollinger–Ellison syndrome in two patients in 1955, there have been significant advances in the understanding of its patho-genesis, natural history, relationship to multiple endocrine neoplasia type 1, diagnosis, methods of tumour localization and management. The main focus in treatment is now shifting from management of the gastric acid hyper-secretory state which can now be controlled medically in almost every patient, to the management of the gastrinoma. Recent studies are beginning to provide insights into the natural history of gastrinomas, factors that are associated with invasiveness in some gastrinomas, defining the role of surgery in managing patients with different disease extents, or with MEN 1 and being able to provide insights into molecular abnormalities that may be important in their pathogenesis. In this article each of these advances is briefly reviewed with emphasis primarily on recent advances.

REFERENCES

Anthony L, Johnson D, Hande K et al (1993) Somatostatin analogue phase I trials in neuroendocrine neoplasms. *Acta Oncologica* **32:** 217–223.
Anthuber M, Jauch KW, Briegel J et al (1996) Results of liver transplantation for gastroentero-pancreatic tumor metastases. *World Journal of Surgery* **20:** 73–76.

Lyons J, Landis CA, Harsh G et al (1990) Two G protein oncogenes in human endocrine tumors. *Science* **249**: 655–659.

MacFarlane MP, Fraker DL, Alexander HR et al (1995) A prospective study of surgical resection of duodenal and pancreatic gastrinomas. *Surgery* **118**: 973–980.

Malagelada J, Edis AJ, Adson MA et al (1983) Medical and surgical options in the management of patients with gastrinoma. *Gastroenterology* **84**: 1524–1532.

Maton PN (1989) The use of the long-acting somatostatin analogue, octreotide acetate, in patients with islet cell tumors. *Gastroenterology Clinics of North America* **18**: 897–922.

Maton PN & Dayal Y (1991) Clinical implications of hypergastrinemia. In Zakim D & Dannenberg AJ (eds) *Peptic Ulcer Disease and Other Acid-Related Disorders*, pp 213–246. Armonk, NY: Academic Research Associates.

Maton PN, Frucht H, Vinayek R et al (1988) Medical management of patients with Zollinger–Ellison syndrome who have had previous gastric surgery: a prospective study. *Gastroenterology* **94**: 294–299.

Maton PN, Gardner JD & Jensen RT (1986) Cushing's syndrome in patients with Zollinger–Ellison syndrome. *New England Journal of Medicine* **315**: 1–5.

Maton PN, Gardner JD & Jensen RT (1989a) Use of the long-acting somatostatin analog, SMS 201–995 in patients with pancreatic islet cell tumors. *Digestive Diseases and Sciences* **34**: 28S–39S.

Maton PN, Mackem SM, Norton JA et al (1989b) Ovarian carcinoma as a cause of Zollinger–Ellison syndrome. Natural history, secretory products and response to provocative tests. *Gastroenterology* **97**: 468–471.

Maton PN, Lack EE, Collen MJ et al (1990) The effect of Zollinger–Ellison syndrome and omeprazole therapy on gastric oxyntic endocrine cells. *Gastroenterology* **99**: 943–950.

McArthur KE, Richardson CT, Barnett CC et al (1996) Laparotomy and proximal gastric vagotomy in Zollinger–Ellison syndrome: results of a 16-year prospective study. *American Journal of Gastroenterology* **91**: 1104–1011.

McCarthy DM (1978) Report on the United States experience with cimetidine in Zollinger–Ellison syndrome and other hypersecretory states. *Gastroenterology* **74**: 453–458.

McCarthy DM (1980) The place of surgery in the Zollinger–Ellison syndrome. *New England Journal of Medicine* **302**: 1344–1347.

McCarthy DM, Olinger EJ, May RJ et al (1977) H_2-histamine receptor blocking agents in the Zollinger–Ellison syndrome. Experience in seven cases and implications for long-term therapy. *Annals of Internal Medicine* **87**: 668–675.

McEntee GP, Nagorney DM, Kvols LK et al (1990) Cytoreductive hepatic surgery for neuroendocrine tumors. *Surgery* **108**: 1091–1096.

McGuigan JE & Trudeau WL (1968) Immunochemical measurement of elevated levels of gastrin in the serum of patients with pancreatic tumors of the Zollinger–Ellison variety. *New England Journal of Medicine* **278**: 1308–1313.

Metz DC & Jensen RT (1995) Advances in gastric antisecretory therapy in Zollinger–Ellison syndrome. In Mignon M & Jensen RT (eds) *Endocrine Tumors of the Pancreas: Recent Advances in Research and Management. Frontiers of Gastrointestinal Research*, vol. 23 pp 240–257. Basel: S. Karger.

Metz DC, Kuchnio M, Fraker DL et al (1993a) Flow cytometry and Zollinger–Ellison syndrome: relationship to clinical course. *Gastroenterology* **105**: 799–813.

Metz DC, Pisegna JR, Fishbeyn VA et al (1993c) Control of gastric acid hypersecretion in the management of patients with Zollinger–Ellison syndrome. *World Journal of Surgery* **17**: 468–480.

Metz DC, Pisegna JR, Ringham GL et al (1993d) Prospective study of efficacy and safety of lansoprazole in Zollinger–Ellison syndrome. *Digestive Diseases and Sciences* **38**: 245–256.

Metz DC, Strader DB, Orbuch M et al (1993d) Use of omeprazole in Zollinger–Ellison: a prospective nine-year study of efficacy and safety. *Alimentary Pharmacology and Therapeutics* **7**: 597–610.

Metz DC, Jensen RT, Bale AE et al (1994) Multiple endocrine neoplasia type 1: clinical features and management. In Bilezekian JP, Levine MA & Marcus R (eds) *The Parathyroids*, pp 591–646. New York: Raven Press.

Metz DC, Weber HC, Orbuch M et al (1995) *Helicobacter pylori* infection: a reversible cause of hypergastrinemia and hyperchlorhydria which can mimic Zollinger–Ellison syndrome. *Digestive Diseases and Sciences* **40**: 153–159.

Mignon M, Ruszniewski P, Haffar S et al (1986) Current approach to the management of tumoral process in patients with gastrinoma. *World Journal of Surgery* **10**: 703–710.

Mignon M, Cadiot G, Rigaud D et al (1995a) Management of islet cell tumors in patients with multiple endocrine neoplasia type 1. In Mignon M & Jensen RT (eds) *Endocrine Tumors of the Pancreas: Recent Advances in Research and Management. Frontiers of Gastrointestinal Research*, vol. 23, pp 342–359. Basel: S. Karger.

Mignon M, Jais P, Cadiot G et al (1995b) Clinical features and advances in biological diagnostic criteria for Zollinger–Ellison syndrome. In Mignon M & Jensen RT (eds) *Endocrine Tumors of the Pancreas: Recent Advances in Research and Management. Frontiers of Gastrointestinal Research*, vol. 23, pp 223–239. Basel: S. Karger.

Miller LS, Vinayek R, Frucht H et al (1990) Reflux esophagitis in patients with Zollinger–Ellison syndrome. *Gastroenterology* **98**: 341–346.

Miller LS, Doppman J, Maton PN et al (1991) Zollinger–Ellison syndrome. Advances in diagnosis and treatment. *Handbook of Experimental Pharmacology* **99**: 349–400.

Miller DL, Doppman JL, Metz DC et al (1992) Zollinger–Ellison syndrome: technique, results and complications of portal venous sampling. *Radiology* **182**: 235–241.

Moertel CG, Hanley JA & Johnson LA (1980) Streptozotocin alone compared with streptozotocin plus fluorouracil in the treatment of advanced islet-cell carcinoma. *New England Journal of Medicine* **303**: 1189–1194.

Moertel CG, Kvols LK, O'Connell MJ & Rubin J (1991) Treatment of neuroendocrine carcinomas with combined etoposide and cisplatin. Evidence of major therapeutic activity in the anaplastic variants of these neoplasms. *Cancer* **68**: 227–232.

Moertel CG, Lefkopoulo M, Lipsitz S et al (1992) Streptozotocin–doxorubicin, streptozotocin–flourouracil or chlorozotocin in the treatment of advanced islet cell carcinoma. *New England Journal of Medicine* **326**: 519–523.

Moertel CG, Johnson CM, McKusick MA et al (1994) The management of patients with advanced carcinoid tumors and islet cell carcinomas. *Annals of Internal Medicine* **120**: 302–309.

Mukai K, Grotting JC, Greider MH & Rosai J (1982) Retrospective study of 77 pancreatic endocrine tumors using the immunoperoxidase method. *American Journal of Surgical Pathology* **6**: 387–399.

Nagorney DM & Que FG (1995) Cytoreductive hepatic surgery for metastatic gastrointestinal neuro-endocrine tumors. In Mignon M & Jensen RT (eds) *Endocrine Tumors of the Pancreas: Recent Advances in Research and Management. Frontiers of Gastrointestinal Research*, vol. 23 pp 416–430. Basel: S. Karger.

Neuburger P, Lewin M, Recherche CD & Bonfils S (1972) Parietal and chief cell population in four cases of the Zollinger–Ellison syndrome. *Gastroenterology* **63**: 937–942.

Norton JA (1994) Advances in the management of Zollinger–Ellison syndrome. *Advances in Surgery* **27**: 129–159.

Norton JA (1995) Surgical treatment of islet cell tumors with special emphasis on operative ultrasound. In Mignon M & Jensen RT (eds) *Endocrine Tumors of the Pancreas: Recent Advances in Research and Management. Frontiers of Gastrointestinal Research*, vol. 23 pp 309–332. Basel: S. Karger.

Norton JA & Jensen RT (1991) Unresolved surgical issues in the management of patients with the Zollinger–Ellison syndrome. *World Journal of Surgery* **15**: 151–159.

Norton JA, Doppman JL, Collen MJ et al (1986a) Prospective study of gastrinoma localization and resection in patients with Zollinger–Ellison syndrome. *Annals of Surgery* **204**: 468–479.

Norton JA, Sugarbaker PH, Doppman JL et al (1986b) Aggressive resection of metastatic disease in selected patients with malignant gastrinoma. *Annals of Surgery* **203**: 352–359.

Norton JA, Cornelius MJ, Doppmann JL et al (1987) Effect of parathyroidectomy in patients with hyperparathyroidism, Zollinger–Ellison syndrome and multiple endocrine neoplasia type I: a prospective study. *Surgery* **102**: 958–966.

Norton JA, Cromack DT, Shawker TH et al (1988) Intraoperative ultrasonographic localization of islet cell tumors. A prospective comparison to palpation. *Annals of Surgery* **207**: 160–168.

Norton JA, Doppman JL & Jensen RT (1992) Curative resection in Zollinger–Ellison syndrome: results of a 10-year prospective study. *Annals of Surgery* **215**: 8–18.

Norton JA, Levin B & Jensen RT (1993) Cancer of the endocrine system. In DeVita VT Jr, Hellman S & Rosenberg SA (eds) *Cancer: Principles and Practice of Oncology*, 4th edn. pp 1333–1435. Philadelphia PA: J.B. Lippincott.

Oberg K (1993) The use of chemotherapy in the management of neuroendocrine tumors. *Endocrinology and Metabolism Clinics of North America* **22**: 941–952.

Oberg K (1994) Expression of growth factors and their receptors in neuroendocrine gut and pancreatic tumors, and prognostic factors for survival. *Annals of the New York Academy of Sciences* **733**: 46–55.

Oberhelman HA Jr, Nelsen TS, Johnson AN & Dragstedt LR (1961) Ulcerogenic tumors of the duodenum. *Annals of Surgery* **153**: 214–227.

Orbuch M, Doppman JL, Strader DB et al (1995) Imaging for pancreatic endocrine tumor localization: recent advances. In Mignon M & Jensen RT (eds) *Endocrine Tumors of the Pancreas: Recent Advances in Research and Management. Frontiers of Gastrointestinal Research*, vol. 23 pp 268–281. Basel: S. Karger.

Perry LJ, Stuart K, Stokes KR & Clouse ME (1994) Hepatic arterial chemoembolization for metastatic neuroendocrine tumors. *Surgery* **116**: 1111–1117.

Pipeleers-Marichal M, Somers G, Willems G et al (1990) Gastrinomas in the duodenums of patients with multiple endocrine neoplasia type 1 and the Zollinger–Ellison syndrome. *New England Journal of Medicine* **322**: 723–727.

Pisegna JR, Norton JA, Slimak GG et al (1992) Effects of curative resection on gastric secretory function and antisecretory drug requirement in the Zollinger–Ellison syndrome. *Gastroenterology* **102**: 767–778.

Pisegna JR, Doppman JL, Norton JA et al (1993a) Prospective comparative study of ability of MR imaging and other imaging modalities to localize tumors in patients with Zollinger–Ellison syndrome. *Digestive Diseases and Sciences* **38**: 1318–1328.

Pisegna JR, Slimak GG, Doppman JL et al (1993b) An evaluation of human recombinant alpha interferon in patients with metastatic gastrinoma. *Gastroenterology* **105**: 1179–1183.

Polacek MA & Ellison EH (1966) Parietal cell mass and gastric acid secretion in the Zollinger–Ellison syndrome. *Surgery* **60**: 606–614.

Que FG, Nagorney DM, Batts KP et al (1995) Hepatic resection for metastatic neuroendocrine carcinomas. *American Journal of Surgery* **169**: 36–43.

Raufman JP, Collins SM, Pandol SJ et al (1983) Reliability of symptoms in assessing control of gastric acid secretion in patients with Zollinger–Ellison syndrome. *Gastroenterology* **84**: 108–113.

Rehfeld JF & Bardram L (1995) Prohormone processing and pancreatic endocrine tumors. In Mignon M & Jensen RT (eds) *Endocrine Tumors of the Pancreas: Recent Advances in Research and Management. Frontiers of Gastrointestinal Research*, vol. 23 pp 84–98. Basel: S. Karger.

Rehfeld JF & van Solinge WW (1994) The tumor biology of gastrin and cholecystokinin. *Advances in Cancer Research* **63**: 295–347.

Reubi JC, Laissue J, Waser B et al (1994) Expression of somatostatin receptors in normal, inflamed, and neoplastic human gastrointestinal tissues. *Annals of the New York Academy of Sciences* **733**: 122–137.

Richardson CT, Peters MN, Feldman M et al (1985) Treatment of Zollinger–Ellison syndrome with exploratory laparotomy, proximal gastric vagotomy, and H_2-receptor antagonists. A prospective study. *Gastroenterology* **89**: 357–367.

Routley D, Ramage JK, McPeake J et al (1995) Orthotopic liver transplantation in the treatment of metastatic neuroendocrine tumors of the liver. *Liver Transplant Surgery* **1**: 118–121.

Ruszniewski P, Hochlas S, Rougier P & Mignon M (1991) Intravenous chemotherapy with streptozotocin and 5-fluorouracil for hepatic metastases of Zollinger–Ellison syndrome. A prospective multicenter study in 21 patients. *Gastroenterology and Clinical Biology* **15**: 393–398.

Ruszniewski P, Podevin P, Cadiot G et al (1993a) Clinical, anatomical, and evolutive features of patients with the Zollinger–Ellison syndrome combined with type I multiple endocrine neoplasia. *Pancreas* **8**: 295–304.

Ruszniewski P, Rougier P, Roche A et al (1993b) Hepatic arterial chemoembolization in patients with liver metastases of endocrine tumors. A prospective phase II study in 24 patients. *Cancer* **71**: 2624–2630.

Ruszniewski P, Amouyal P, Amouyal G et al (1995a) Localization of gastrinomas by endoscopic ultrasonography in patients with Zollinger–Ellison syndrome. *Surgery* **117**: 629–635.

Ruszniewski P, Amouyal P, Amouyal G et al (1995b) Endocrine tumors of the pancreatic area: localization by endoscopic ultrasonography. In Mignon M & Jensen RT (eds) *Endocrine Tumors of the Pancreas: Recent Advances in Research and Management. Frontiers of Gastrointestinal Research*, vol. 23 pp 258–267. Basel: S. Karger.

Saeed ZA, Norton JA, Frank WO et al (1989) Parenteral antisecretory drug therapy in patients with Zollinger–Ellison syndrome. *Gastroenterology* **96**: 1393–1402.

Saltz L, Trochanowski B, Buckley M et al (1993) Octreotide as an antineoplastic agent in the treatment of functional and nonfunctional neuroendocrine tumors. *Cancer* **72**: 244–248.

Sawicki MP, Wan YJ, Johnson CL et al (1992) Loss of heterozygosity on chromosome 11 in sporadic gastrinomas. *Human Genetics* **89**: 445–449.

Scarpignato C (1995) Somatostatin analogues in the management of endocrine tumors of the pancreas. In Mignon M & Jensen RT (eds) *Endocrine Tumors of the Pancreas: Recent Advances in Research and Management. Frontiers of Gastrointestinal Research.* vol. 23 pp 385–414. Basel: S. Karger.

von Schrenck T, Howard JM, Doppman JL et al (1988) Prospective study of chemotherapy in patients with metastatic gastrinoma. *Gastroenterology* **94**: 1326–1334.

Shepherd JJ, Challis DR, Davies PF et al (1993) Multiple endocrine neoplasm, type 1: gastrinomas, pancreatic neoplasms, microcarcinoids, the Zollinger–Ellison syndrome, lymph nodes, and hepatic metastases. *Archives of Surgery* **128**: 1133–1142.

Skogseid B & Oberg K (1995) Genetics of multiple endocrine neoplasia type 1. In Mignon M & Jensen RT (eds) *Endocrine Tumors of the Pancreas: Recent Advances in Research and Management. Frontiers of Gastrointestinal Research,* vol. 23 pp 60–69. Basel: S. Karger.

Solcia E, Capella C, Sessa F et al (1986) Gastric carcinoids and related endocrine growths. *Digestion* **35 (supplement 1):** 3–22.

Solcia E, Bordi C, Creutzfeldt W et al (1988) Histopathological classification of nonantral gastric endocrine growths in man. *Digestion* **41**: 185–200.

Solcia E, Capella C, Fiocca R et al (1989) The gastroenteropancreatic endocrine system and related tumors. *Gastroenterology Clinics of North America* **18**: 671–693.

Solcia E, Capella C, Fiocca R et al (1990) Gastric argyrophil carcinoidosis in patients with Zollinger–Ellison syndrome due to type 1 multiple endocrine neoplasia. A newly recognized association. *American Journal of Surgical Pathology* **14**: 503–513.

van Solinge WW, Odum L & Rehfeld JF (1993) Ovarian cancers express and process progastrin. *Cancer Research* **53**: 1823–1828.

Stadil F (1995) Treatment of gastrinomas with pancreatoduodenectomy. In Mignon M & Jensen RT (eds) *Endocrine Tumors of the Pancreas: Recent Advances in Research and Management. Frontiers of Gastrointestinal Research,* vol. 23 pp 333–341. Basel: S. Karger.

Stokes KR, Stuart K & Clouse ME (1993) Hepatic arterial chemoembolization for metastatic endocrine tumors. *Journal of Vascular Interventional Radiology* **4**: 341–345.

Strader DB, Doppman JL, Orbuch M et al (1995) Functional localization of pancreatic endocrine tumors. In Mignon M & Jensen RT (eds) *Endocrine Tumors of the Pancreas: Recent Advances in Research and Management. Frontiers of Gastrointestinal Research,* vol. 23 pp 282–297. Basel: S. Karger.

Stremple JF & Meade RC (1968) Production of antibodies to synthetic human gastrin I and radioimmunoassay of gastrin in the serum of patients with the Zollinger–Ellison syndrome. *Surgery* **64(1):** 165–174.

Sugg SL, Norton JA, Fraker DL et al (1993) A prospective study of intraoperative methods to diagnose and resect duodenal gastrinomas. *Annals of Surgery* **218**: 138–144.

Syversen U, Mignon M, Bonfils S et al (1993) Chromogranin A and pancreastatin-like immunoreactivity in serum of gastrinoma patients. *Acta Oncologica* **32**: 161–165.

Thom AK, Norton JA, Axiotis CA & Jensen RT (1991) Location, incidence and malignant potential of duodenal gastrinomas. *Surgery* **110**: 1086–1093.

Thom AK, Norton JA, Doppman JL et al (1992) Prospective study of the use of intraarterial secretin injection and portal venous sampling to localize duodenal gastrinomas. *Surgery* **112(6):** 1002–1008.

Thompson JC, Lewis BG, Wiener I & Townsend CM Jr (1983) The role of surgery in the Zollinger–Ellison syndrome. *Annals of Surgery* **197(5):** 594–607.

Thompson NW, Czako PF, Fritts LL et al (1994) Role of endoscopic ultrasonography in the localization of insulinomas and gastrinomas. *Surgery* **116**: 1131–1138.

Ur E, Bomanji J, Mather SJ et al (1993) Localization of neuroendocrine tumours and insulinomas using radiolabelled somatostatin analogues, ^{123}I-Tyr^3-octreotide and ^{111}In-pentatreotide. *Clinical Endocrinology* **38**: 501–506.

Vessey SJR, Jones PM, Wallis SC et al (1994) Absence of mutations in the Gsα and Gi2α genes in sporadic parathyroid adenomas and insulinomas. *Clinical Science* **87**: 493–497.

Vinayek R, Frucht H, London JF et al (1990) Intravenous omeprazole in patients with Zollinger–Ellison syndrome undergoing surgery. *Gastroenterology* **99**: 10–16.

spiral CT appears to represent a significant advance over previous technology, we plan to evaluate it in an investigational setting. The combination of IOUS and careful surgical palpation has allowed us to cure 97.4% of benign insulinomas and we feel justified in avoiding other pre-operative tests with their associated time, invasiveness and expense. Because the focus of interest and expertise differs among institutions, however, and technical advances continue to occur, there is no single 'correct' answer. A balance must be struck between routine exhaustive, expensive pre-operative imaging and inadequate localization efforts that may contribute to frequent, even more expensive surgical failures.

SURGICAL MANAGEMENT

Pre-operative preparation

When a diagnosis has unequivocally been established, and appropriate localization procedures completed, operative treatment is planned. The patient is admitted to hospital the evening before the operation, an intravenous catheter is placed and a 10% solution of dextrose is infused overnight to avoid any risk of hypoglycaemia. Approximately 2–3 hours prior to beginning the operation, we discontinue the glucose infusion and allow modest hypoglycaemia to develop. The glucose level is expected to fall gradually during the course of the operation under close monitoring. Limited if any bowel preparation is necessary because the need to enter the bowel is exceptionally uncommon. A pre-operative dose of prophylactic antibiotics may be administered.

Intraoperative management

We continue to utilize intraoperative blood glucose monitoring, expecting a progressive rise within minutes to an hour of insulinoma resection (Tutt et al, 1980). However, a lack of the rebound hyperglycaemia should not by itself instigate additional resection, as a delay in the response may occur in over 20% of patients. We do not allow the glucose to drop below 40–50 mg/dl, depending on the patient's pre-operative glucose levels and clinical symptoms at low glucose levels.

Technique

A bilateral subcostal incision with the use of a fixed retracting device under the costal margins gives excellent exposure to the entire upper abdomen. Initial exploration includes careful assessment of the liver for metastatic disease.

The pancreas is exposed by dissecting the omentum from the transverse colon throughout its entire length. The omentum and stomach are retracted superiorly, lysing congenital adhesions between the posterior wall of the stomach and the pancreas. If pre-operative localization has identified the site of the tumour, the next efforts should be directed accordingly. The head of the pancreas is mobilized by a generous Kocher manoeuvre, carrying the posterior dissection medially over the aorta, and around the second and third portions of the duodenum, opening the plane between it and the hepatic flexure of the colon. If the neck of the pancreas must be widely exposed, the gastroepiploic artery and vein (as it joins the gastro-colic venous trunk which empties into the superior mesenteric vein (SMV) at the inferior border of the pancreas) can be safely sacrificed. The SMV can be exposed by following the middle colic vein superiorly, then mobilized from the adjacent head and uncinate process of the pancreas by transecting the inferior pancreaticoduodenal vein. The body and tail of the pancreas are mobilized by incising the peritoneum at the inferior border of the gland, and gradually dissecting beneath its entire posterior surface. The spleen may be mobilized, and transecting the short gastric and gastroepiploic vessels will allow the pancreas to be lifted completely out of the left upper quadrant. Care must be exercised in avoiding damage to

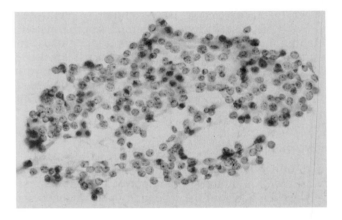

Figure 5A.

Figure 5. Intraoperative ultrasound identified a non-palpable insulinoma immediately adjacent to the ampulla, adjacent to the duodenum. (A) With IOUS guidance, a fine-needle aspiration (FNA) was obtained and the smear shows a sheet of small, granular islet cells, indicative of insulinoma. (B) On the basis of the IOUS image of the tumour and the FNA result, a pancreatoduodenectomy was performed and the tumour is seen in the middle of the bisected pancreatic specimen.

Figure 6. Most times when multiple insulinomas are encountered, the disease is MEN 1 related. This patient, however, with three large tumours in the distal body and tail of the pancreas had only sporadic disease, with no other endocrinopathies.

Figure 8. Mobilized pancreas of a young female patient with multiple insulinomas typical of her disease, MEN 1.

Figure 9. Pancreatoduodenectomy of a malignant insulinoma illustrating the white, desmoplastic tumour invading into surrounding normal pancreatic parenchyma and duodenum.

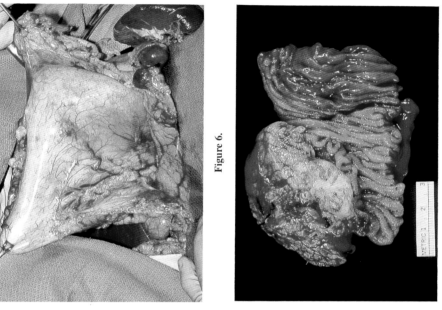

Figure 6.

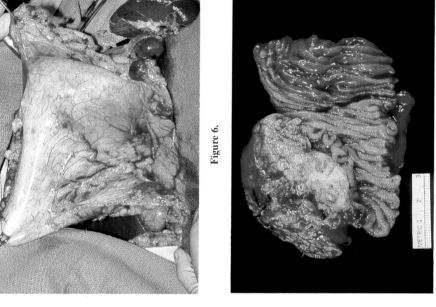

Figure 9.

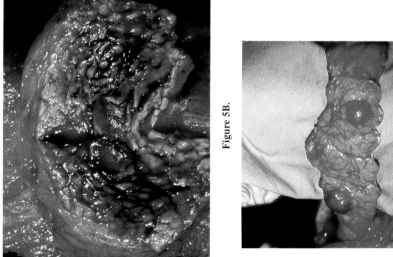

Figure 5B.

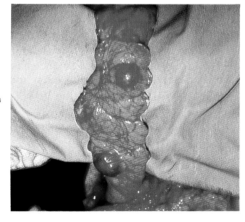

Figure 8.

the underlying left adrenal gland. Following completion of all of these steps, the pancreas will be completely exposed. Gentle bidigital palpation of the entire gland will permit nearly 90% of tumours to be identified. Uncommonly, the reddish-purple or white tumours are actually exposed on the surface, but rather they are typically covered by a layer of pancreatic parenchyma.

Unless the tumour has been identified on the edge of the pancreas, well out of danger from any anatomical structure, primarily the pancreatic duct, a radiologist scrubs in at this point to perform IOUS. The entire pancreas is surveyed to assist in locating a tumour or to exclude additional tumours (Figure 6) if one has already been identified. The pancreatic duct and any other relevant anatomical structures are identified and their relationships to the tumour are carefully defined. In this way, the safest approach to the tumour can be planned, and the location of the pancreatic duct can be anticipated if it must be dissected from the tumour surface.

Our preferred method of removing insulinomas is by enucleation. Insulinomas almost always have a pseudocapsule and a clear dissection plane between the compact tumour and the softer, characteristic normal pancreatic parenchyma. If the tumour is hard, causes puckering of surrounding soft tissue, appears to be infiltrating, or causing distal dilatation of the pancreatic duct, one must be highly suspicious of a malignancy, and resection rather than enucleation must be chosen. The tumour is enucleated by dissecting immediately adjacent to the tumour, bluntly separating the tumour from normal pancreas using fine instruments and a small sucker. This is facilitated by using the left-hand fingers behind the gland, and the thumb anteriorly to provide countertraction on the tumour. If the tumour is firm, a stitch can be placed through the tumour to lift it and to provide additional traction. Once the tumour has been enucleated, rather than risk trauma to the surrounding normal pancreas by closing the defect with sutures, I often leave it open, or instill fibrin glue into it. Almost always a drain is left near the defect.

When the tumour is anatomically unsuitable for enucleation, resection of the distal pancreas is a safe and effective alternative. The spleen is preserved when possible. Again, the cut edge of the pancreas is drained, even if the main pancreatic duct has been specifically closed with stitches or clips, and fibrin glue has been applied. In our practice, since 1980, only two benign insulinomas in the head of the pancreas have required a Whipple resection (Table 2).

Results

We have been successful in identifying, excising, and returning patients to euglycaemia in 111 of 114 (97.4%) patients with benign insulinomas from 1980 to 1995. The three who were not cured include one patient with MEN 1 syndrome, who had five tumours identified and enucleated from the pancreas, but modest hypoglycaemia recurred within 2 months. One patient, who underwent resection for a combination of nesidioblastosis and insulin-producing adenomas, was not cured. Re-exploration did not reveal any additional tumours. She is well controlled on verapamil. No tumour was found in the last patient who takes diazoxide with adequate control. Our 97.4% success rate compares favourably with others reported in the literature, ranging from 77% to 100% (Rothmund et al, 1990; Doherty et al, 1991; Menegaux et al, 1992).

No tumour identified, re-operation

In contrast to former years, following introduction of the localization techniques of THPVS and IOUS, few authors now advocate sequential blind distal pancreatic resections when no tumour is identified. Because at least 50% of palpably occult insulinomas are located in the head or uncinate process of the pancreas, distal pancreatectomy would be destined to failure. Moreover, completion pancreatectomy carries potentially serious consequences; in a review from our institution, among nine patients undergoing total pancreatectomy for insulinoma, there was one operative death and seven of the remaining patients died prematurely from complications related to the apancreatic state (Thompson et al, 1993). Fortunately, this has not been required since 1981.

When an insulinoma has not been identified at the first operation, and re-operation is contemplated, referral to a centre with considerable experience is mandatory. Some have advocated using medical therapy until pre-operative localization has been achieved (Kaplan, 1989). The diagnosis must be reconfirmed, potentially extensive pre-operative localization may be required, and surgical re-exploration is often significantly more difficult. The dissection planes are scarred and the pancreas is firmer, compromising one's ability to palpate the tumour. Nevertheless, since the introduction of IOUS in our practice, 10 of 11 re-operative patients have been cured by enucleating (Figure 7) the tumours (Thompson et al, 1993). The only patient not cured is the patient with nesidioblastosis.

Complications

Despite gentle, careful, precise technique, the addition of IOUS, and the occasional use of perioperative somatostatin, an operation on the pancreas can still yield complications. They can be divided into those related and unrelated to the actual pancreatic procedure. Nine patients (8%) developed complications unrelated to the pancreatic dissection, comprising acute myocardial infarction, congestive heart failure, paroxysmal atrial tachycardia, partial omental torsion and infarction, wound infection, acute appendicitis, *Clostridium dificile* diarrhoea, bile duct obstruction, and bleeding from a Dieulefoy's lesion of the stomach. Pancreatic complications included abscess, pseudocyst, or fistula formation, and occurred in 14 (12%) patients. There was no post-operative mortality in this series, and none since 1941 at the Mayo Clinic.

In other large series, pancreatic-related complications have occurred in

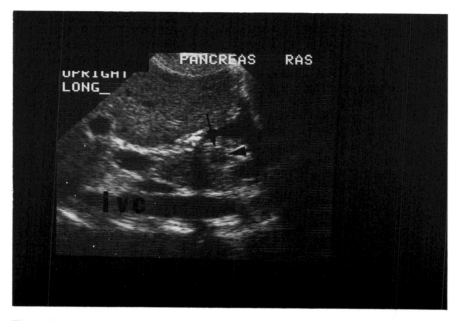

Figure 7. Intraoperative ultrasound image of the head of the pancreas in an 18 year old male who had undergone unsuccessful exploration and distal pancreatectomy 5 years prior to this exploration. The tumour (arrows) is demonstrated at the level of the inferior vena cava (ivc).

16% (Doherty et al, 1991) to 43% (Menegaux et al, 1992) of patients. Perhaps with more frequent use of IOUS with clear delineation of the anatomical relationship of the pancreatic duct to the tumour, these rates will decline.

Post-operative management

Throughout the operative procedure, no glucose is given intravenously unless the level has dropped below 40–50 mg/dl. We continue withholding glucose in the IV fluids for an additional 24 hours. During this time, the glucose level often rises to 180–230 mg/dl. If a significant portion of pancreas has been resected, the peak level may exceed 250 mg/dl in which case we will often give small doses of insulin. We maintain surveillance of the glucose level utilizing reflectance meter measurements approximately three times daily initially; this is then reduced to a single morning fasting glucose measurement by the time of hospital discharge.

We do not routinely use somatostatin prophylactically or continue antibiotics beyond the first day. The drain adjacent to the pancreas is removed once the patient is tolerating a general diet and the drainage is minimal, usually within 7 days post-operatively.

Patients who have undergone splenectomy are given vaccinations against meningococcus and *H. influenza*, and Pneumovax the day prior to hospital dismissal to diminish the risk of post-splenectomy sepsis (Schwartz et al, 1982).

MEDICAL MANAGEMENT

Dietary management

Most commonly effective and used in the medical management of insulinoma is dietary therapy. Frequent meals or snacks designed to avoid prolonged periods of time without glucose intake may suffice. Complex carbohydrates as prophylaxis, and readily available forms of glucose, for example orange juice, for symptoms of hypoglycaemia are recommended. Implantable glucose pumps for continuous glucose infusion may be necessary to control refractory hypoglycaemia resulting from malignancy.

Diazoxide

The most commonly used drug in the medical management of hyper-insulinism is diazoxide, a well-known antihypertensive agent with hyper-glycaemic effects. It suppresses insulin secretion by direct action on the β cells and also works through an extrapancreatic effect by enhancing glycogenolysis (Fajans et al, 1968). In the usual therapeutic dose of 200–600 mg p.o. daily, it offers reasonably good control of hyperglycaemia in approximately 50% of patients (Goode et al, 1986). Unfortunately, oedema, weight gain, and hirsutism complicate an equal number of patients, and nausea occurs in over 10%. While some have advocated a trial of this medication prior to surgical exploration when pre-operative localization has been unproductive (Goode et al, 1986), we utilize it only in patients following failed exploration or in those with unresectable metastatic or diffuse disease.

Calcium channel blockers

Our experience using verapamil to control the hyperglycaemia in one patient with combined nesidioblastosis and insulin-producing adenomas has been impressive. The drug has also been used successfully in other patients with insulinoma (Murakami et al, 1979; De Marinis and Barbarino, 1980; Ulbrecht et al, 1986).

Somatostatin analogue

In our experience as well as that of others (Fajans and Vinik, 1989), synthetic somatostatin analogue has yielded only temporary and modest relief of hypoglycaemia.

Angiographic ablation

Angiographic ablation of an insulinoma by embolization has been reported (Moore et al, 1982), but would seem of only limited value owing to the rich anastomotic blood supply of the pancreas.

SPECIAL SITUATIONS

Multiple endocrine neoplasia I syndrome

Multiple endocrine neoplasia type I is an autosomal dominant disease characterized by endocrinopathies of the parathyroid glands, the anterior pituitary, and the endocrine pancreas. The genetic origin was first described by Wermer (1963) and later the gene was mapped to chromosome 11 (Larsson et al, 1988). Whereas the pancreatic islet cell tumours overall are most frequently gastrin secreting, the dominant functioning tumour in patients under the age of 25 is insulinoma (Shepherd, 1991).

Between 1970 and 1991, 19 patients with MEN 1 syndrome underwent surgical treatment for insulinoma at the Mayo Clinic (O'Riordain et al, 1994). A single patient had unresectable malignancy, but 16 (89%) of the remaining 18 patients had multicentric benign disease (Figure 8). Cure of hypoglycaemia was achieved in 17 of the 18 patients, and recurrence only occurred in the patients in whom conservative pancreatic resection was performed. Distal subtotal pancreatic resection to approximately the level of the portal vein, with enucleation of tumours in the head of the pancreas whenever possible, proved to be excellent treatment. With over 10 years of follow-up, only a single patient was not cured, as a result of unresected tumours remaining in the head of the gland. Malignant disease was identified in two patients, one with unresectable disease, referred to previously, and a second patient (10.5%) with a single nodal micrometastasis. No patient had a duodenal tumour resected for insulinoma in contrast to gastrinomas in the MEN syndrome (Thompson et al, 1989).

Evolving from analysis of the Mayo Clinic data as well as an extensive review by Demeure et al (1991), the surgical strategy must be guided by the almost universal tumour multiplicity and consequent disease recurrence in the absence of aggressive initial resection. Total gross tumour removal plus adequate prophylactic resection to minimize the risk of recurrent hyperglycaemia, yet to prevent endocrine and exocrine pancreatic insufficiency, is the fine balance that must be struck in these patients. Routine distal pancreatectomy with enucleation of tumours in the head of the gland, guided by IOUS for safe removal, achieves these goals. Little is to be gained by pre-operative localization imaging given this plan.

Malignancy

Malignant insulinomas are rare, accounting for about 5–10% of all insulinomas (Service et al, 1991). By definition, these tumours must show evidence of local invasion into surrounding soft tissue or metastasis (to the liver or nodes) to be considered malignant (Figure 9). Cytological changes alone are not adequate to classify a tumour as malignant, and attempts to use nuclear DNA ploidy and cell cycle analysis have not proved valuable in distinguishing benign from malignant islet-cell tumours (Stipa et al, 1987; Graeme-Cook et al, 1990). In addition, reports of elevated levels of chorionic gonadotropin (Kahn et al, 1977) and its subunits and a high percentage of proinsulin have correlated with malignancy. However, a proinsulin level greater than 60% was found in five of 16 benign insulinomas in one report (Pasieka et al, 1992), and nine of 25 in another (Doherty et al, 1991), negating the value of this measurement.

Patients with malignant insulinoma have the same clinical manifestations as those with benign disease, namely symptoms of hypoglycaemia. Because metastases also maintain hormonal hypersecretion, only complete resection will alleviate the symptoms completely. Danforth et al (1984) reviewed the literature in 1984 and found only 62 cases of metastatic insulinoma. The tumours were usually single and large, averaging 6 cm in diameter. The median disease-free survival after curative resection was 5 years, but recurrence occurred in 63% of cases at a median interval of 2.8 years, followed by a median survival with recurrent tumour of only 19 months. Palliative resection yielded a median survival of 4 years, but biopsy only 11 months. They recommended aggressive attempts at resection as these tumours are less virulent than their malignant ductal counterparts. Ten-year survival of 29% has been reported in malignant insulinomas (Service et al, 1991).

Cytoreductive hepatic surgery for metastatic insulinoma has rarely been reported but, for the combination of islet-cell tumours and carcinoids, experience with 74 patients would suggest that hepatic resection can be performed with less than a 3% mortality, provide effective palliation, and probably prolong survival (Que et al, 1995). It appears that if all disease can be removed, surgical resection is optimal. Palliative resection should be considered only when at least 90% of the tumour bulk can be excised (McEntee et al, 1990).

When surgical options have been exhausted, medical management as previously described should be considered. Additionally, chemotherapy in the form of adriamycin and streptozocin has been associated with a 69% tumour regression rate, and remission from endocrine symptoms has extended to 18 months (Moertel et al, 1992). Unfortunately, this combination of drugs is also associated with considerable toxicity.

SUMMARY

Fundamental to establishing a diagnosis of insulinoma is first to consider the diagnosis when presented with the constellation of symptoms and signs that indicate hypoglycaemia. Prominent and most convincing are manifestations of neuroglycopenia. Although hypoglycaemia can be caused by a number of disorders, the combination of hypoglycaemia and endogenous hyperinsulinaemia is diagnostic of insulinoma. Our criteria now include a glucose level of 40 mg/dl with a concomitant insulin level of 6 µU/ml, a C-peptide level exceeding 200 pmol/l, and negative screen for sulphonlyurea. Ancillary diagnostic tests or the use of insulin surrogates may offer helpful confirmation. Localization is still evolving, but in our hands pre-operative ultrasound is the best and only pre-operative test that we obtain in the usual situation. Expertise and experience with other modalities at other institutions offer reasonable but more costly alternatives. Intraoperative ultrasonography provides significant benefit in both tumour localization and delineating important related anatomy. Insulinomas are virtually all located in the pancreas; 90% are benign, single, and are generally firmer than surrounding normal pancreas. Extensive exposure may be required to identify and remove safely the tumour. Enucleation is our preferred technique, but distal pancreatectomy for tumours in the body or tail is an excellent method as well. Pancreatoduodenectomy is rarely necessary. Complications most commonly relate to leak of pancreatic secretions, causing pseudocyst, abscess, or fistula. Except in MEN 1 syndrome, excision of a benign insulinoma equates with disease cure, and patients are often extraordinarily grateful as the change in their lives may be profound.

REFERENCES

Angelini L, Bezzi M, Tucci G et al (1987) The ultrasonic detection of insulinomas during surgical exploration of the pancreas. *World Journal of Surgery* **11:** 642–647.

Archambeaud-Mouveroux F, Huc MC, Nadalon S et al (1989) Autoimmune insulin syndrome. *Biomedical Pharmacotherapy* **43:** 581–586.

Banting FG & Best CH (1922) The internal secretion of the pancreas. *Journal of Laboratory and Clinical Medicine,* **7:** 251–266.

Block MB, Gambetta M, Resnekov L et al (1972) Spontaneous hypoglycaemia in congestive heart-failure. *Lancet* **2:** 736–738.

Bressler R, Corredor C & Brendel K (1969) Hypoglycin and hypoglycin-like compounds. *Pharmacology Review* **21:** 105–130.

Cho KJ, Vinik AI, Thompson N et al (1982) Localization of the source of hyperinsulinism. *American Journal of Roentgenology* **139:** 237–245.

Dagget PR, Goodburn EA, Kurtz AB et al (1981) Is preoperative localisation of insulinomas necessary? *Lancet* **i:** 483.

Danforth DN Jr, Gorden P & Brennan MF (1984) Metastatic insulin-secreting carcinoma of the pancreas: clinical course and the role of surgery. *Surgery* **96:** 1027–1036.

Daughaday WH (1989) Hypoglycemia in patients with non-islet cell tumors. *Endocrinology and Metabolism Clinics of North America* **18:** 91–101.

De Marinis L & Barbarino A (1980) Calcium antagonists and hormone release. I. Effects of verapamil on insulin release in normal subjects and patients with islet-cell tumor. *Metabolism* **29:** 599–604.

Delcore R & Friesen SR (1994) Gastrointestinal neuro endocrine tumors. *Journal of the Americal College of Surgeons* **178:** 187–211.

Demeure MJ, Klonoff DC, Karam JH et al (1991) Insulinomas associated with multiple endocrine neoplasia type I: the need for a different surgical approach. *Surgery* **110:** 998–1005.

Doherty GM, Doppman JL, Shawker TH et al (1991) Results of a prospective strategy to diagnose, localize, and resect insulinomas. *Surgery* **110:** 989–997.

Doppman JL, Miller DL, Chang R et al (1991) Insulinomas: localization with selective intra-arterial injection of calcium. *Radiology* **178:** 237–241.

Dunnick NR, Long J & Krudy A (1980) Localizing insulinomas with combined radiographic methods. *American Journal of Roentgenology* **135:** 747–752.

Fajans SS & Vinik AI (1989) Insulin-producing islet cell tumors. *Endocrinology and Metabolism Clinics of North America* **18:** 45–74.

Fajans SS, Floyd JC Jr & Thiffault CA (1968) Further studies on diazoxide suppression of insulin release from abnormal and normal islet tissue in man. *Annals of the New York Academy of Science* **150:** 261–280.

Felig P, Brown WV, Levine RA et al (1970) Glucose homeostasis in viral hepatitis. *New England Journal of Medicine* **283:** 1436–1440.

Felig P, Cherif A, Minagawa A et al (1982) Hypoglycemia during prolonged exercise in normal men. *New England Journal of Medicine* **306:** 895–900.

Fletcher A & Campbell W (1922) The blood sugar following insulin administration and the symptom complex-hypoglycemia. *Journal of Metabolism Research* **2:** 637.

Fulton RE, Sheedy PT & McIlrath DC (1975) Preoperative angiographic localization of insulin-producing tumors of the pancreas. *American Journal of Roentgenology* **123:** 367–377.

Garber AJ, Bier DM, Cryer PE et al (1974) Hypoglycemia in compensated chronic renal insufficiency: substrate limitation of gluconeogenesis. *Diabetes* **23:** 982–986.

Glaser B, Shapiro B, Fajrans S & Vinik AI (1988) Effects of secretin on the normal and pathologic beta cell. *Journal of Clinical Endocrinology and Metabolism* **66:** 1138–1144.

Glickman MH, Hart MJ & White TT (1980) Insulinoma in Seattle: thirty-nine cases in 30 years. *American Journal of Surgery* **140:** 119–125.

Goode PN, Farndon JR, Anderson J et al (1986) Diazoxide in the management of patients with insulinoma. *World Journal of Surgery* **10:** 586–592.

Goodenow TJ & Malarkey WB (1977) Leukocytosis and artifactual hypoglycemia. *Journal of the American Medical Association* **237:** 1961–1962.

Gordon P & Roth J (1969) Plasma insulin: fluctuations in the 'big' insulin component in man after glucose and other stimuli. *Journal of Clinical Investigation* **48:** 2225–2234.

Gower WR & Fabri PJ (1990) Endocrine neoplasms (non-gastrin) of the pancreas. *Seminars in Surgical Oncology* **6:** 98–109.

Graeme-Cook F, Bell DA, Flotte TJ et al (1990) Aneuploidy in pancreatic insulinomas does not predict malignancy. *Cancer* **66:** 2365–2368.

Grama D, Eriksson B, Mårtensson H et al (1992) Clinical characteristics, treatment and survival in patients with pancreatic tumors causing hormonal syndromes. *World Journal of Surgery* **16:** 632–639.

Grant CS, van Heerden JA, Charboneau JW et al (1988) Insulinoma: the value of intraoperative ultrasonography. *Archives of Surgery* **123:** 843–848.

Heard CRC (1978) The effects of protein-energy malnutrition on blood glucose homeostasis. *World Review of Nutrition Dietetics* **30:** 107–147.

Hogan MJ, Service FJ, Sharbrough FW et al (1983) Oral glucose tolerance test compared with a mixed meal in the diagnosis of reactive hypoglycemia: a caveat on stimulation. *Mayo Clinic Proceedings* **58:** 491–496.

Howland G, Campbell WR, Maltby EJ et al (1929) Dysinsulinism: convulsions and coma due to islet cell tumor of the pancreas with operation and cure. *Journal of the American Medical Association* **93:** 674.

Kahn RC, Rosen SW, Weintraub BD et al (1977) Ectopic production of chorionic gonadotropin and its subunits by islet-cell tumors: a specific marker for malignancy. *New England Journal of Medicine* **297:** 565–569.

Kaplan EL (1989) Insulinoma: surgical and diagnostic approach. In van Heerden JA (ed.) *Common Problems in Endocrine Surgery*, pp 272–281. Chicago, IL: Year Book Medical Publishers.

Klotter JJ, Ruckert K, Kummerle F et al (1987) The use of intraoperative sonography in endocrine tumors of the pancreas. *World Journal of Surgery* **11:** 635–641.

Kojak G Jr, Barry MJ Jr & Gastineau CF (1969) Severe hypoglycemic reaction with haloperidol: report of a case. *American Journal of Psychiatry* **126:** 573–576.

Laidlaw GF (1938) Nesidioblastosis in adults: a surgical dilemma. *American Journal of Pathology* **14:** 125.

Laroche GP, Ferris DO & Priestley JT (1968) Hyperinsulinism. *Archives of Surgery* **96:** 765–772.

Larsson C, Skogseid B, Oberg K et al (1988) Multiple endocrine neoplasia type I gene maps to chromosome 11 and is lost in insulinoma. *Nature* **332:** 85.

Lev-Ran A & Anderson RW (1981) The diagnosis of postprandial hypoglycemia. *Diabetes* **30:** 996–999.

Levin H & Heifetz M (1990) Phaeochromocytoma and severe protracted postoperative hypoglycaemia. *Canadian Journal of Anaesthesiology* **37**: 477–478.

Limburg PJ, Katz H, Grant CS et al (1993) Quinine-induced hypoglycemia. *Annals of Internal Medicine* **119**: 218–219.

Luyckx AS & LeFebvre PJ (1971) Plasma insulin in reactive hypoglycemia. *Diabetes* **20**: 435–442.

Madison LL (1968) Ethanol-induced hypoglycemia. *Advances in Metabolic Disorders*, 3: 85–109.

Marks V & Teale JD (1991) Tumours producing hypoglycaemia. *Diabetes and Metabolism Reviews* **7**: 79–91.

McEntee GP, Nagorney DM, Kvols LK et al (1990) Cytoreductive hepatic surgery for neuroendocrine tumors. *Surgery* **108**: 1091–1096.

Menegaux F, Schmitt G, Mercadier M et al (1992) Pancreatic insulinomas. *American Journal of Surgery* **165**: 243–248.

Miller SI, Wallace RJ Jr, Musher DM et al (1980) Hypoglycemia as a manifestation of sepsis. *American Journal of Medicine* **68**: 649–654.

Moertel CG, Lefkopoulo M & Lipsitz S (1992) Streptozocin–doxorubicin, streptozocin–fluorouracil, or chlorozotocin in the treatment of advanced islet-cell carcinoma. *New England Journal of Medicine* **326**: 519–523.

Moore TJ, Peterson LM, Harrington DP et al (1982) Successful arterial embolization of an insulinoma. *Journal of the American Medical Association* **248**: 1353–1357.

Murakami K, Taniguchi H, Kobayashi T et al (1979) Suppression of insulin release by calcium antagonist in human insulinoma *in vivo* and *in vitro:* its possible role for clinical use. *Kobe Journal of Medical Science* **25**: 237–247.

Nicholls AG (1902) Simple adenoma of the pancreas arising from an island of Langerhans. *Journal of Medical Research* **8**: 385.

Norton JA, Shawker TH, Doppman JL et al (1990) Localization and surgical treatment of occult insulinomas. *Annals of Surgery* **212**: 615–620.

O'Riordain DS, O'Brien T, van Heerden JA et al (1994) Surgical management of insulinoma associated with multiple endocrine neoplasia type I. *World Journal of Surgery* **18**: 488–494.

Pasieka JL, McLeod M, Thompson NW et al (1992) Surgical approach to insulinomas; assessing the need for preoperative localization. *Archives of Surgery* **127**: 442–447.

Que FG, Nagorney DM, Batts KP et al (1995) Hepatic resection for metastatic neuroendocrine carcinomas. *American Journal of Surgery*, **169**: 36–43.

Robbins DC, Tager HS & Rubenstein AH (1984) The biologic and clinical importance of proinsulin. *New England Journal of Medicine* **310**: 165–175.

Roche A, Raisonnier A & Gillon-Savouret M-C (1982) Pancreatic venous sampling and arteriography in localizing insulinomas and gastrinomas: procedure and results in 55 cases. *Radiology*, **145**: 621–627.

Roche T, Lightdale CJ & Botet JF (1992) Localization of pancreatic endocrine tumors by endoscopic ultrasonography. *New England Journal of Medicine* **326**: 1721–1726.

Rothmund M, Angelini L & Brunt M (1990) Surgery for benign insulinoma: an international review. *World Journal of Surgery* **14**: 393–399.

Rynearson EH (1947) Hyperinsulinism among malingerers. *Medical Clinics of North American* **31**: 477.

Schwartz, PE, Sterioff S, Mucha P et al (1982) Post splenectomy sepsis and mortality in adults. *Journal of the American Medical Association* **248**: 2279–2283.

Service FJ (1992) Factitial hypoglycemia. *Endocrinologist* **2**: 173–176.

Service FJ (1995) Hypoglycemic disorders. *New England Journal of Medicine* **332**: 1144–1152.

Service FJ, Dale AJD, Elveback LR et al (1976) Insulinoma: clinical and diagnostic features of 60 consecutive cases. *Mayo Clinic Proceedings*, **51**: 417–429.

Service, FJ, McMahon MM, O'Brien PC et al (1991) Functioning insulinoma—incidence, recurrence, and long-term survival of patients: a 60-year study. *Mayo Clinic Proceedings* **66**: 711–719.

Service FJ, O'Brien PC, Kao PC et al (1992) C-peptide suppression test: effects of gender, age, and body mass index; implications for the diagnosis of insulinoma. *Journal of Clinical Endocrinology and Metabolism* **74**: 240–210.

Shepherd JJ (1991) The natural history of multiple endocrine neoplasia type I: highly uncommon or highly unrecognized? *Archives of Surgery* **126**: 935.

Starr JI & Rubenstein AH (1974) Metabolism of endogenous proinsulin and insulin in man. *Journal of Clinical Endocrinology and Metabolism* **38**: 305–307.

Stefanini P, Carboni M & Patrassi N (1974) Beta-islet cell tumors of the pancreas: results of a study on 1,067 cases. *Surgery* **75:** 597–609.

Stipa F, Arganini M, Bibbo M et al (1987) Nuclear DNA analysis of insulinomas and gastrinomas. *Surgery* **102:** 988–998.

Talente GM, Coleman RAJ & Alter C (1994) Glycogen storage disease in adults. *Annals of Internal Medicine* **120:** 218–226.

Taylor SI, Grunberger G, Marcus-Samuels B et al (1982) Hypoglycemia associated with antibodies to the insulin receptor. *New England Journal of Medicine* **307:** 1422–1426.

Thompson NW, Vinik AI & Eckhauser FE (1989) Microgastrinomas of the duodenum. *Annals of Surgery* **209:** 396–404.

Thompson GB, Service FJ, van Heerden JA et al (1993) Reoperative insulinomas, 1927 to 1992: an institutional experience. *Surgery* **114:** 1196–1206.

Tutt G Jr, Edis AJ, Service FJ et al (1980) Plasma glucose monitoring during operation for insulinoma: a critical reappraisal. *Surgery* **88:** 351–356.

Ulbrecht JS, Schmeltz R & Aarons JH (1986) Insulinoma in a 94-year-old woman: long-term therapy with verapamil. *Diabetes Care* **9:** 186–188.

van Heerden JA & Edis AJ (1980) Insulinoma: diagnosis and management. *Surgical Rounds* **3:** 42–51.

van Heerden JA & Edis AJ & Service FJ (1979) The surgical aspects of insulinomas. *Annals of Surgery* **189:** 677–682.

Wermer P (1963) Endocrine adenomatosis and peptic ulcer in a large kindred. *American Journal of Medicine* **35:** 205.

Whipple AO & Franz VK (1935) Adenoma of islet cells with hyperinsulinism. *American Surgeon* **101:** 1299–1335.

Wilder RM, Allan FN, Power MH et al (1927) Carcinoma of the islets of the pancreas: hyperinsulinism and hypoglycemia. *Journal of the American Medical Association* **89:** 348–355.

Yakovac WC, Baker L & Hummeler K (1971) Beta cell nesidioblastosis in idiopathic hypoglycemia of infancy. *Journal of Pediatrics* **79:** 226.

Zimmerman BR (1983) Hypoglycemia from hepatic, renal and endocrine disorders. In Service FJ (ed.) *Hypoglycemia: Pathogenesis, Diagnosis, and Treatment.* Boston, MA: G.K. Hall.

6

Vasoactive intestinal polypeptide-secreting tumours: biology and therapy

SANG KYU PARK
M. SUE O'DORISIO
THOMAS M. O'DORISIO

Vasoactive intestinal polypeptide (VIP) secreting tumours (VIPomas) are rare tumours arising from the VIP-secreting cells of the gastrointestinal tract or nervous system.

The association of pancreatic islet cell tumours and diarrhoea was first reported by Priest and Alexander (1957) but was considered a variant of the Zollinger–Ellison syndrome. Verner and Morrison (1958) described two patients with profuse watery diarrhoea, hypokalaemia and achlorhydria associated with a non-β islet cell pancreatic adenocarcinoma. Elevated levels of VIP were first reported in the plasma and tumours from patients with this diarrhoeogenic syndrome by Bloom et al (1973).

VIPomas occur in pancreatic (90%) and extrapancreatic (10%) sites. Most extrapancreatic VIPomas occur along the autonomic nervous system and in the adrenal medulla as neuroblastomas, ganglioneuromas or ganglio-neuroblastomas (Mitchell et al, 1976; Jansen-Goemans and Engelhardt, 1977; Long et al, 1981a). The precise cellular origin of this tumour remains controversial, but a neural crest origin is suggested because of the neuro-transmitter action of VIP (Capella et al, 1983). Extrapancreatic VIPomas arising in the retroperitoneum, lungs, oesophagus, jejunum and liver have also been reported (Said and Faloona, 1975; Capella et al, 1983; Watson et al, 1985).

This chapter will discuss VIP-secreting pancreatic tumours, liver tumours and neuroblastic tumours.

VIP-SECRETING PANCREATIC TUMOURS

Epidemiology and anatomy

VIPomas account for 2–7% of gastroenteropancreatic (GEP) neuro-endocrine tumours (Krejs, 1987; Debas and Mulvihill, 1994) and have a reported annual incidence of 1 per 10 million population (Krejs, 1987). The

Baillière's Clinical Gastroenterology—
Vol. 10, No. 4, December 1996
ISBN 0–7020–2186–5
0950–3528/96/040673 + 24 $12.00/00

mean age of patients is 49 years (range 32–75 years), and there appears to be a slight preponderance of women (54%) (Long et al, 1981a).

Pancreatic VIPomas are usually solitary (70–80%) with an average diameter of 1–7 cm (maximum reported, 20 cm) (Rothmund et al, 1991), and much more commonly located in the body and tail (75%) than in the head (25%) of the pancreas (Mozell et al, 1990). In various series, 37–68% of the VIPomas were metastatic to the liver, regional lymph nodes, kidneys, lungs, stomach or mediastinum at the time of diagnosis or surgery (Verner and Morrison, 1974; Long et al, 1981a; Capella et al, 1983). In one detailed study, 61% of VIPomas were identified as malignant, which is comparable with the 63–90% malignancy rate reported with gastrinomas, glucagonomas and somatostatinomas (Capella et al, 1983).

Pathology and pathophysiology

Capella et al (1983) summarized and discussed the clinical, biochemical, histological, histochemical and ultrastructural findings in 32 VIPomas (31 pancreatic and one jejunal). All cases showed light microscopic features of epithelial tumours including trabecular and tubuloacinar structures and reactivity with Grimelius' silver stain. Mitoses were uncommon, seen in only 12%. On electron microscopy a mixture of cells was seen, usually in the same tumour, with 90% having cells with a few scattered, inconspicuous secretory granules, and 52% having some well-differentiated endocrine cells with small, well-developed granules.

Most secretory granules were round, small (120–180 nm diameter) and of moderate electron density, resembling those of the so-called D1 cells of the normal human pancreas and gut. According to immunocytochemical analysis, VIP was detected in 86% of VIPomas. Most VIPomas also synthesize at least one other neuropeptide, such as pancreatic polypeptide (PP) (39%), somatostatin (14%), insulin (14%), glucagon (7%) and neurotensin (7%). Calcitonin (Yamaguchi et al, 1980), α-chain of human chorionic gonadotrophin (Yagihashi et al, 1982), methionine-enkephalin (Yagihashi et al, 1982; Solcia et al, 1988), and chromogranin B (Woussen-Colle et al, 1995) also have been detected in pancreatic VIPomas. Neither the histological studies nor the electron microscopic studies allow VIPomas to be clearly differentiated from some other pancreatic endocrine tumours; however, the presence of immunoreactive VIP is strongly suggestive of VIPoma, as this is uncommonly found in other pancreatic endocrine tumours (10 of 104 in one study) (Heitz et al, 1982).

It is now clear that VIP is the major mediator of the VIPoma syndrome (Krejs, 1987; O'Dorisio et al, 1989). For a number of years there was considerable controversy about the mediator (Krejs, 1987). Receptors for VIP have been identified on intestinal epithelial cells (Laburthe and Amiranoff, 1989). The three major types of effects of VIP that may be physiological in the gut are the relaxation of smooth muscle, vasodilation and stimulation of exocrine pancreatic and intestinal secretion (Walsh and Mayer, 1993). The most important aspect of VIP action relating to symptomatology in patients is that of a potent intestinal secretagogue. VIP

octreotide, which has a half-life of nearly 3 days and is excreted renally, was developed (Krenning et al, 1992); this has recently been approved for use in the United States for the imaging of primary and metastatic gastro-enteropancreatic neuroendocrine tumours and lymphomas. Joseph et al (1993) showed that receptor scintigraphy with [^{111}In]DTPA-D-Phe^1-octreotide is a simple method with a sensitivity of 86% for the localization of the primary tumour and its metastases in patients presenting with the clinical and biochemical symptoms of an endocrine tumour of the gastro-intestinal tract or the pancreas. In 85 patients with GEP tumours, receptor scintigraphy proved to be superior to ultrasound and CT in 34%, equal in 52% and inferior in 14% of the cases. Positive somatostatin scintigraphy correlates well with in vitro somatostatin receptor and predicts response to octreotide therapy (Figure 1). Recently, VIP itself has been shown to be a promising imaging agent. Virgolini et al (1994) were able to localize in vivo, the tumours of patients with gastrointestinal neuroendocrine tumours. Receptor-based scintigraphy may be of greatest value in identifying the extent of metastatic disease; it is an excellent diagnostic tool for identi-fication of extra-abdominal spread, particularly to lymph nodes, lungs and bone (Hammond et al, 1994).

Receptor-based scintigraphy is likely to be of limited value in identify-ing small primary VIPomas of 0.3–0.5 cm diameter (Joseph et al, 1992; Hammond et al, 1994). However, these small tumours may be clinically very significant. Schirmer et al (1993) have utilized radioreceptor-guided surgery to localize small primary tumours in the operating room. A small dose of [^{125}I]Tyr^3-octreotide was injected 2–24 hours prior to surgery; in the operating room, a hand-held γ-detecting probe was used to detect in situ tumour binding of the radioiodinated somatostatin-analogue. This surgical technique has successfully located occult primary tumours, even when all other conventional imaging methods have failed. An example of the time course of uptake of the radiolabelled somatostatin analogue in a VIPoma as recorded during surgery is shown in Figure 2. Indeed, this patient experienced a 'VIPoma crisis' on manipulation of the tumour. The ensuing profound hypotension and vascular collapse were corrected within 2 minutes with intravenous octreotide acetate therapy.

Treatment (Table 2)

Supportive therapy

Correction of fluid and electrolyte deficits is critical in patients with signs and symptoms of VIPoma. Initial treatment for the WDS is the replacement of large fluid losses (often exceeding 9 litres/day), the correction of hypo-kalaemia and the reversal of acidosis. The oral administration of glucose electrolyte solutions and potassium supplements may suffice in correcting the fluid deficits in mild cases. More severe cases usually require hospital-ization for intensive intravenous fluid replacement, potassium supple-mentation of as much as 400 mEq/day and meticulous correction of other electrolyte and acid–base abnormalities. The magnitude and route of

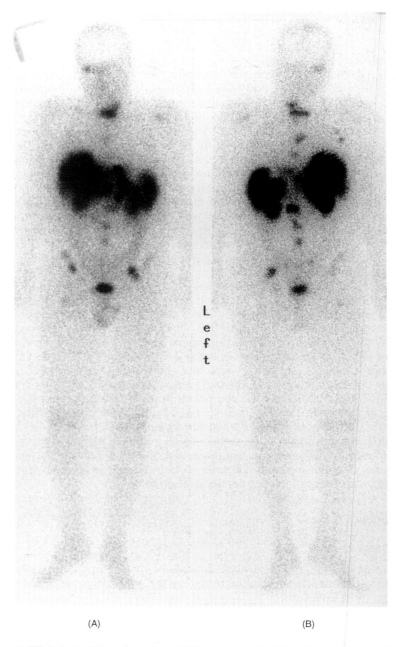

(A)   (B)

Figure 1. Whole-body, 24 hour, OctreoScan® ([¹¹¹In]pentetreotide). OctreoScan of a 48-year-old male
with metastatic VIPoma syndrome: (A) anterior view; (B) posterior view. Note adequacy of scan as
demonstrated by visualization of thyroid. Striking extra abdominal lesions are noted, as well as skull,
pelvic and thoracic cavity lesions.

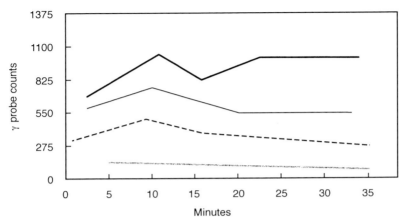

Figure 2. Radioreceptor-guided surgery identification of VIPoma intra-operatively. A time course of an intra-operative radiolabelled peptide ([^{125}I]Tyr^3-octreotide) guided surgery in a 72 year old male with metastatic VIPoma syndrome is depicted. On the vertical axis are γ counts per 2 seconds; time in minutes is shown on the horizontal axis. The uppermost tracing indicates γ counts from the liver tumour; these counts are higher than normal liver, normal aorta and normal bowel. Histopathology confirmed tumour as VIPoma. ▬▬, = tumour; ───, = liver; - - -, = aorta; ∼∼∼, = bowel, normal.

administration of fluid therapy can be individualized, depending on the severity of the diarrhoea and the degree of the patient's electrolyte imbalance (O'Dorisio et al, 1989; Miller et al, 1990).

Pharmacotherapy

Somatostatin is a potent inhibitor of human exocrine pancreatic secretion and has the advantage of suppressing both hormone release and hormone action for several peptides produced by endocrine tumours (Debas and Gittes, 1993). Somatostatin has been shown in a wide variety of experimental preparations to inhibit VIP-induced intestinal anion secretion and to stimulate sodium chloride absorption (Carter et al, 1978; Dharmsathaphorn et al, 1980a,b; Freedman et al, 1980; Guandalini et al, 1980; Rosenthal et al, 1983). The broad potential spectrum of clinical applications is limited by the short serum half-life of only 3 minutes and the fact that somatostatin must be given intravenously. This problem with natural somatostatin has been overcome with the recent development of octreotide.

A cyclic somatostatin derivative, octreotide has been used to treat secretory diarrhoea associated with VIPoma. The central active moiety of the somatostatin molecule consists of the four amino acids Phe, D-Trp, Lys and Thr which are mandatory for the biological action of somatostatin. Octreotide contains this essential part of the molecule stabilized by a disulphide bond and extended by the two amino acids Phe and Thr which prevent the immediate degradation characteristic of natural somatostatin

Table 2. Therapy of VIPomas.

Modality	Comment
Supportive therapy	
Intravenous fluids	Severe cases may require > 6 litres/day
Intravenous electrolytes	Correct profound hypokalaemia (often > 350 mEq K^+/day)
	Correct hypomagnesaemia
	Correct metabolic acidosis
Somatostatin or somatostatin analogues	First-line symptomatic therapy; somatostatin analogues (octreotide, lanreotide and octastatin) are effective in the symptomatic improvement of the WDS in > 90% of VIPoma patients
Surgery	Considered as both initial therapy and, when possible, debulking therapy; radioreceptor-guided surgery using [^{125}I]octreotide helpful in localization of occult primary and metastatic foci
Pharmacotherapy	All other modalities should be considered only in the
Glucocorticoids	patients who have failed to respond to a trial of
Indomethacin	clinically available somatostatin analogues
Lithium carbonate	
Clonidine	
Angiotensin II	
Norepinephrine	
Carbonate phenothiazine	
Phosphate buffer	
Metaclopromide	
Loperamide	
Chemotherapy	Combination therapy is useful but does not produce
Streptozotocin	permanent remission. Renal and hepatic impairment
5-Fluorouracil	from some drugs can be very serious and usually drug
Chlorozotocin	limiting
DTIC	
Human leukocyte interferon	
Adriamycin	
Immunotherapy	
Monoclonal anti-tumour antibodies	Need further studies

and other gastrointestinal peptides (Arnold et al, 1994). It has a long enough half-life (90 minutes) and a duration of action of 8 hours to be given subcutaneously only one to three times a day (Bauer et al, 1982). Currently, octreotide or other long-acting somatostatin congeners such as lantreotide and octastatin are the therapeutic principle of choice in suppressing the release of hormones from endocrine GEP tumours. These analogues also have a direct action at the target cell itself, thus also preventing water and electrolyte secretion. These two actions together improve the characteristic clinical symptomatology in nearly all patients with functional endocrine GEP tumours. In more than 25 patients with VIPoma in the literature treated with octreotide, the characteristic watery diarrhoea, typically unresponsive to other agents, was completely controlled in 56% of patients and significantly improved in another 28%. Plasma VIP levels fell by about

60%. Indeed, octreotide is the most effective known drug therapy for this disease (Debas and Gittes, 1993).

The mechanism by which somatostatin inhibits diarrhoea in VIPoma is dual and based on the inhibition of hormone release–synthesis from the tumour and by the direct inhibition of water and electrolyte secretion from the intestine (Ruskone et al, 1982). Yasunami et al (1994) isolated human VIPoma cells from the resected specimen of a pancreatic tumour from a patient with WDS. VIPoma cells released VIP and PP simultaneously; carbachol stimulated the release of both VIP and PP, which was abolished by the addition of atropine. Phorbol myristate acetate (PMA), a protein kinase C activator, also stimulated VIP and PP release similarly to carbachol, suggesting that the cells have a muscarinic receptor that mediates VIP and PP release. Octreotide has a direct inhibitory effect on the VIP and PP release stimulated by carbachol and PMA. Fassler et al (1990) demonstrated that octreotide inhibited increases in short-circuit current (I_{sc}) induced by VIP, serotonin and substance P. Octreotide significantly inhibited the intestinal secretory response to all the secretagogues studied, at the level of the intestinal epithelial cell.

This dual action may explain why, in many patients receiving octreotide, plasma VIP concentration falls, but in only 30% of treated patients does it approach normal levels while the diarrhoea remains controlled. A marked discrepancy exists in the literature concerned with the anti-tumour effect in the VIPomas. A review by Dunne et al (1989) failed to demonstrate any predictable anti-tumour activity of octreotide on the tumour size, growth or progression of metastatic disease. This is contrary to other studies indicating that somatostatin analogue may cause tumour regression in patients with metastatic VIPoma (Clements and Elias, 1985; Kraenzlin et al, 1985). Additionally, there is some evidence that octreotide can change the chromatographic elution pattern with VIPoma, indicating that it may alter its biological activity (Anderson and Bloom, 1986). However, individual patients show considerable variation in clinical response to octreotide, making it necessary to titrate dose to achieve optimal control of symptoms. A consensus development panel which was held in May 1993 established guidelines for octreotide dose titration in patients with secretory diarrhoea (Harris et al, 1995).

In VIPoma patients, the initial dose and subsequent titration regimen depend on the condition of the patient. Patients with life-threatening symptoms, such as severe metabolic acidosis, hypokalaemia, hypercalcaemia, hypotension, shock or profound secretory diarrhoea, should be given a 100 mg bolus intravenously followed by 50 mg/hour intravenously until stable. The route of octreotide administration can then be changed to subcutaneous in patients responding satisfactorily. For patients with milder symptoms, an initial dose of 100–150 mg subcutaneously every 8 hours is recommended. Patients' stool output and electrolyte status should be monitored on a daily or weekly basis, depending on symptom severity. If the response to the initial dose is insufficient, octreotide administration should be increased in 50 mg increments per dose, up to 200 mg every 8 hours. If needed, the dose can be further increased in 100 mg increments per dose, from 200 mg to a maximum of 500 mg every 8 hours. Once control has been attained and symptoms have been adequately suppressed for at least 2–3 weeks, the dose may be titrated down to the minimum level required for control by decreasing the dose per injection by 25 mg on a weekly basis. Administration of dexamethasone may prevent tachyphylaxis to octreotide and permit continuous use of octreotide at a similar or lower dose. The end-point of treatment should focus on a reduction of diarrhoea rather than normalization of hormone profile (Harris et al, 1995).

Adverse effects with octreotide therapy have been remarkably few. Pain is experienced at the injection site because of the acid pH of the solution. Some abdominal cramping, bloating, flatulence, nausea and vomiting may be seen initially but this subsides with time. Hyperglycaemia and abnormal glucose tolerance are seen with more frequency but are of little clinical significance. Of much greater importance is the rare hypoglycaemic reaction. The latter side-effect is seen in the first 24–48 hours of therapy and tends to occur in catabolic patients. Transient elevations in serum transaminase have also been reported. With long-term therapy, particularly with high doses, pancreatic exocrine insufficiency and steatorrhoea develop. This is well controlled with oral pancreatic enzyme replacement. Faecal fat measurements serve as a good guide to replacement therapy. Pancreatic exocrine insufficiency occurs because of the inhibition of the release and action of cholecystokinin (CCK) as well as a direct inhibitory action of octreotide on acinar cell function. Similarly, octreotide therapy results in the inhibition of gall-bladder contraction that can be demonstrated by ultrasonography. Indeed, 20–25% of patients on long-term octreotide therapy will develop gallstones. This complication should be monitored using periodic ultrasound imaging (Debas and Gittes, 1993).

Before the development of octreotide, glucocorticoids constituted the mainstay of medical management of VIP-induced diarrhoea. They have been reported to produce a 40–50% reduction in VIP levels both in vitro and in vivo (Mekhjian and O'Dorisio, 1987). The mechanism by which steroids improve diarrhoea may involve enhanced sodium absorption in the small or large intestine and also inhibition of VIP release from the tumour. Methylprednisone induces the synthesis of Na^+/K^+-ATPase and has been shown to decrease cholera-induced intestinal secretion (Charney and Donowitz, 1976). Doses in the range from 60 to 80 mg (prednisone equivalent) should be employed. Many other pharmacological agents have been employed in the management of VIPoma-induced diarrhoea. Indomethacin, a prostaglandin inhibitor, has been reported to decrease stool volume with an oral dose of 25 mg every 8 hours (Jaffe et al, 1977; Albuquerque et al, 1979). Lithium carbonate at 300 mg twice a day is reported to decrease stool volume despite continued high plasma VIP levels (Pandol et al, 1980). The mechanism may be due to cAMP inhibition. Other agents include clonidine (McArthur et al, 1982), angiotensin II (Rao et al, 1984), norepinephrine (Field and McColl, 1973), carbonate phenothiazines (Donowitz et al, 1980; Smith and Field,

1980), phosphate buffer (VanDyk et al, 1981), metaclopromide (Long et al, 1981b) and loperamide (Yamashiro et al, 1982). However, none of these agents has been studied as extensively or in sufficiently large number of patients to warrant their use as an initial form of therapy. At this time, these agents should be considered only in the patient who has failed to respond to other more-established drug therapies, particularly a trial of octreotide.

Surgery

The most definitive treatment for VIPoma is surgery. The surgical management of pancreatic VIPomas poses a complicated set of questions resulting from their rare occurrence and the difficulty in establishing a diagnosis in early cases or, conversely, the problems inherent in dealing with metastatic disease. However, because their biological behaviour is rather indolent, a real opportunity exists for cure of most patients and for meaningful palliation in patients with extensive metastatic disease (Grant, 1993). Ideally, the patient should be stabilized with regard to haemodynamic and electrolyte abnormalities before any surgical exploration. With the availability of the octreotide, most patients can be managed conservatively during the initial presentation, thus providing the opportunity to investigate the patient for tumour localization. Once the diagnosis is firmly established, abdominal exploration should be undertaken even where pre-operative attempts to locate the lesion have failed. Radioreceptor-guided surgery is of particular benefit in the latter situation.

About 40% of VIPomas are benign and, therefore, are potentially resectable if the diagnosis is made early. Microadenomas or islet cell hyperplasia constitute 20% of tumours, and intra-operative ultrasonography may assist in identifying these small adenomas (Mekhjian and O'Dorisio, 1987). In the past, if no identifiable tumour was found at laparotomy, a 75% distal pancreatectomy was recommended; however, a trial of therapy with a somatostatin analogue would now be appropriate prior to an empirical partial pancreatectomy (Leavey et al, 1995). At the time of exploration, it is important to palpate the adrenal glands and the sympathetic nerve-bearing areas of extrapancreatic neoplasms. Even if all the tumour cannot be removed, surgical debulking results in substantial alleviation of symptoms in approximately 40% of patients, even though the average survival time is 1 year (O'Dorisio and Mekhjian, 1984). Tumour debulking procedures aid both symptomatic management with somatostatin analogues and further reduction of tumour mass by chemotherapy. Metastatic tumours should be aggressively resected, especially if the patient is young and in otherwise good nutritional status. This is justified because these tumours are slow growing, and a reduction of tumour mass can provide long-term symptomatic relief (Miller et al, 1990).

Because of the possibility of rebound gastric-acid hypersecretion and acute peptic ulceration, peri-operative H_2 blocker therapy is recommended (Jaffe, 1987). There can also be a post-operative shift of large volumes of water from the gastrointestinal tract to the intravascular space, resulting in intravascular volume overload. Pre-operative stabilization with octreotide may prevent these complications (Grier, 1995).

Chemotherapy

Clinical trials using cytotoxic chemotherapy in VIPomas have been limited because of the relative rarity of these tumours. Thus, relatively few agents have been systematically studied.

Streptozocin is a chemotherapeutic agent commonly used in the management of pancreas islet cell carcinoma. It is a broad-spectrum antibiotic and a naturally occurring nitrosourea that causes relatively selective destruction of the pancreatic B cell (Modlin et al, 1993).

The combination of 5-fluorouracil (5-FU) and streptozotocin has proved to be effective in approximately 65% of patients enrolled in the Eastern Cooperative Oncology Group and a complete response rate of 33% (Moertel et al, 1980) has been found. The major problem with streptozotocin is distressing gastrointestinal (98%) and renal (65%) toxicity or hepatic toxicity (67%) (Broder and Carter, 1973). Chlorozotocin, which has diminished nephrotoxic and emetic potential compared with streptozotocin, has been shown to produce a similar response rate to streptozotocin alone (Miller et al, 1990) Dimethyltriazino-imidazole-carboxamide (DTIC), human leukocyte interferon and adriamycin in combination with streptozocin have all been used in a small number of patients with variable success (Kessinger et al, 1983; Eriksson et al, 1986). Combination chemotherapy for VIPoma remains relatively unsatisfactory, given the agents currently available. The introduction of newer cytotoxic modalities deserves extensive evaluation (Modlin et al, 1993).

Immunotherapy

Paul et al (1989) described using purified IgG from a human subject to hydrolize VIP in vitro, suggesting a potential immunotherapy for the VIPoma in the future. Monoclonal anti-tumour antibodies have been used for the treatment of various neoplasms, and objective responses with remission of even metastatic lesions have been reported occasionally (Catane and Longo, 1988; Mellstedt et al, 1989). Endocrine tumours may be interesting in this respect, because they often constitute slowly growing neoplasms with the potential to cause pronounced morbidity from an excessive hormone release also in the absence of extensive tumour spread.

Juhlin et al (1994) generated the murine monoclonal antibody of the IgG2$_a$ subtype by immunization with dispersed tumour cells from a pancreatic VIPoma associated with liver and peritoneal metastases as well as a therapy-resistant VIPoma syndrome. Infusion of 100 mg antibody over 2 days into the common hepatic artery of the patient was accompanied by reduced diarrhoea volume until death 6 weeks later. Post-mortem examination demonstrated disappearance of peritoneal metastases as well as absence of immunostaining for the injected antibody and the transferrin receptor within residual hepatic tumour, which constitutes a general marker of proliferating cells (Sutherland et al, 1981). These investigators propose that the short-term effects of a murine monoclonal antibody in VIPoma syndrome should encourage further studies of the therapeutic use of such antibodies in patients harbouring endocrine tumours associated with a pronounced morbidity.

NEUROBLASTIC TUMOUR

In children less than 10 years old and rarely in adults (5% of cases), the VIPoma syndrome is due to tumours along the autonomic chain and in the adrenals (Long et al, 1981a). Histologically, these lesions are ganglio-neuromas, ganglioblastomas or neuroblastomas (Verner and Morrison, 1958; Long et al, 1981a). Long et al (1981a) reported that during a 6-year period (1973–1979) 52 patients with pancreatic tumours and 10 with ganglioneuroblastomas were found to have VIPomas. Metastases were present in only one of the ganglioneuroblastoma patients.

Kimura et al (1993) detected VIP, PHM, neuropeptide Y, methionine-enkephalin, somatostatin, substance P, corticotrophin-releasing hormone and tyrosine hydroxylase in ganglionic cells and some neurites of three ganglioneuroblastomas with WDS. Also the presence of mRNA of VIP or PHM-27, neuropeptide Y, and somatostatin was detectable in the cytoplasm of the tumour cells by in situ hybridization indicating that multiple peptide genes are transcribed and translated simultaneously in these tumours.

Notably, VIP expression has been shown to accompany the histological maturation of neuroblastoma to more benign ganglioneuroblastomatous elements (Mendelsohn et al, 1979). Furthermore, elevated serum levels of VIP correlate with a favourable prognosis in children with neurogenic tumours (Lacey et al, 1989). As such, it has been postulated that VIP may be important in the modulation of neuroblastic growth and differentiation. Pincus et al (1990) demonstrated that VIP can modulate mitosis, differentiation and survival of cultured sympathetic neuroblasts. Studies with neuroblastoma cell lines indicate that, rather than just being a product of partially differentiating malignant cells, VIP plays a role in initiating or promoting differentiation (Pence and Shorter, 1990). Pence and Shorter (1992, 1993) maintained that concomitant enhancement of both intra-cellular and extracellular VIP expression, coupled with the induction of functional specific VIP receptors during VIP-induced differentiation, provides critical evidence for the autocrine regulation of neuroblastoma maturation by peptides. O'Dorisio et al (1992) supported an autocrine function for VIP by studying the VIP receptor and adenylate cyclase activity in neuroblastoma cell lines and primary tumours. Qualman et al (1992) quantified neuropeptide contents in neuroblastomas using radio-immunoassay to assess their possible biological significance. An increased VIP content was correlated with both favourable tumour stage and differentiation. In one composite ganglioneuroblastoma, the ganglio-neuromatous tumour contained nearly a 60-fold greater level of VIP than the level in neuroblastomatous foci. Somatostatin levels similarly were linked to tumour differentiation, suggesting an interactive biological function between VIP and somatostatin in neuroblastoma that may imply a complex multihormonal autocrine growth control mechanism at the cellular level (Muller et al, 1989; O'Dorisio et al, 1992). The WDS associated with VIPomas was not documented in any of these patients with neuroblastomas; this may be related to the existence of various VIP biological forms (Scheibel et al, 1982; Svoboda et al, 1986) or to the coexpression of somatostatin in these tumours (Woltering et al, 1986). Pence and Shorter (1990) also suggest that it is the local tumour content rather than humoral concentration of VIP that may be critical to cellular differentiation in vivo of the tumour, consistent with this peptide's apparent autocrine function.

Pence et al (1994) examined fresh frozen tumour specimens for the presence of VIP and VIP receptors and analysed these results in the light of the known survival data. They concluded that the majority of ganglio-neuroblastomas and a subset of neuroblastomas synthesize immunoreactive VIP in situ. Tumours producing VIP also express an increased number of VIP receptors; VIP synthesis and increased receptor expression correlate with better clinical outcome.

Recent work has already identified another factor that may be important in this system. High serum levels of another neuropeptide, neuropeptide Y, have been identified in association with some cases of neuroblastoma and shown to correlate with an unfavourable prognosis (Hayashi et al, 1991). It is very likely that normal growth and development of sympathetic neuro-blasts will turn out to be under the control of both VIP and neuropeptide Y, with the two having opposing effects.

HEPATIC VIPoma

Since the liver and biliary tree are derived from the foregut anlage together with the ventral pancreas, it is not surprising that endocrine-type tumours have been recorded also in this organ system, both with and without evidence of hormone production (Goodman et al, 1984).

Ayub et al (1993) reported the first case of primary hepatic VIPoma. The 35-year-old male presented with a 3 year history of voluminous watery diarrhoea. Investigations revealed a solitary liver mass and an elevated VIP level. An extensive work-up did not show any other extrahepatic primary lesion. Surgical resection ameliorated all of his symptoms, accompanied by a decrease in the VIP level.

Lundstedt et al (1994) reported two cases of hepatic VIPoma. One patient had a VIPoma syndrome with diarrhoea, hypokalaemia and hyper-calcaemia; all symptoms were reversible after treatment consisting of somatostatin analogue and arterial liver embolization followed by liver resection. The other patient showed no endocrine symptoms.

It has been stressed that extensive search for an extrahepatic tumour must be performed before a neuroendocrine tumour can be accepted as primary in the liver.

Pence JC, Kerns B-JM & Shorter NA (1994) Autocrine regulation of neuroblastoma cell growth and differentiation by vasoactive intestinal peptide. *Advances in Neuroblastoma Research* **4:** 269–274.

Pincus DW, DiCicco-Bloom EM & Black IB (1990) Vasoactive intestinal peptide regulates mitosis, differentiation and survival of cultured sympathetic neuroblasts. *Nature* **343:** 564–567.

Priest WM & Alexander MK (1957) Islet-cell tumor of the pancreas with peptic ulceration, diarrhea and hypokalemia. *Lancet* **ii:** 1145.

Qualman SJ, O'Dorisio MS, Fleshman DJ et al (1992) Neuroblastoma: correlation of neuropeptide expression in tumor tissue with other prognostic factors. *Cancer* **70:** 2005–2012.

Rao MB, O'Dorisio TM, George JM & Gaginella TS (1984) Angiotensin II and norepinephrine antagonize the secretory effect of VIP in rat ileum and colon. *Peptides* **5:** 291–294.

Rood RP, DeLellis RA, Dayal Y & Donowitz M (1988) Pancreatic cholera syndrome due to a vasoactive intestinal polypeptide-producing tumor: further insights into the pathophysiology. *Gastroenterology* **94:** 813–818.

Rosch T, Charles CJ, Botet JF et al (1992) Localization of pancreatic endocrine tumors by endoscopic ultrasonography. *New England Journal of Medicine* **326:** 1721–1726.

Rosenthal LE, Yamashiro DJ, Rivier J et al (1983) Structure–activity relationships of somatostatin analogs in the rabbit ileum and the rat colon. *Journal of Clinical Investigation* **71:** 840–849.

Rothmund M, Stinner B & Arnold R (1991) Endocrine pancreatic carcinoma. *European Journal of Surgical Oncology* **17:** 191–199.

Ruskone A, Rene E, Chayvialle JA et al (1982) Effect of somatostatin on diarrhea and on small intestinal water and electrolyte transport in a patient with pancreatic cholera. *Digestion Disease Science* **27:** 459–466.

Said SI & Faloona GR (1975) Elevated plasma and tissue levels of vasoactive intestinal polypeptide in the watery-diarrhea syndrome due to pancreatic, bronchogenic and other tumors. *New England Journal of Medicine* **293:** 155–160.

Salomon R, Couvineau A, Rouyer-Fessard C et al (1993) Characterization of a common VIP-PACAP receptor in human small intestinal epithelium. *American Journal of Physiology* **264:** E294–E300.

Scheibel E, Rechwitzer C, Fahrenkrug J & Hertz H (1982) Vasoactive intestinal peptide (VIP) in children with neural crest tumors. *Acta Physiologica Scandinavica* **71:** 721–725.

Schiller LR, Rivera LM, Santangelo WC et al (1994) Diagnostic value of fasting plasma peptide concentrations in patients with chronic diarrhea. *Digestion Disease Science* **39:** 2216–2222.

Schirmer WJ, O'Dorisio TM, Schirmer TP et al (1993) Intraoperative localization of neuroendocrine tumors using ^{125}I-tyr(3)-octreotide and a hand-held gamma detecting probe. *Surgery* **3:** 745–752.

Schmitt MG, Soergel KH, Hensley GT & Chey WY (1975) Watery diarrhea associated with pancreatic islet cell carcinoma. *Gastroenterology* **69:** 206–216.

Schwartz SE, Fitzgerald MA, Levine RA & Schwartzel EH (1978) Normal jejunal cyclic nucleotide content in a patient with secretory diarrhea. *Archives of Internal Medicine* **38:** 1403–1405.

Shawker TH, Doppman JL, Dunnick NR & McCarthy DM (1982) Ultrasonic investigation of pancreatic islet cell tumors. *Journal of Ultrasound in Medicine* **1:** 193–200.

Smith PL & Field M (1980) In vitro antisecretory effects of trifluoperazine and other neuroleptics in rabbit and human small intestine. *Gastroenterology* **78:** 1545–1553.

Smitherman TC, Sakio H, Geumei AM et al (1982) Coronary vasodilator action of VIP. In Said SI (ed.) *Vasoactive Intestinal Peptide*, pp 169–176. New York: Raven Press.

Solcia E, Capella C, Riva C et al (1988) The morphology and neuroendocrine profile of pancreatic epithelial VIPomas and extrapancreatic, VIP-producing, neurogenic tumors. *Annals of the New York Academy of Sciences* **527:** 508–517.

Sutherland R, Delia D, Schneider C et al (1981) Ubiquitous cell-surface glycoprotein on tumor cells is proliferation-associated receptor for transferrin. *Proceedings of the National Academy of Sciences of the USA* **78:** 4515–4519.

Svoboda M, Gregoire A, Yanaihara C et al (1986) Identification of two pro-VIP forms in a human neuroblastoma cell line. *Peptides* **7:** 7–15.

Tatemoto K & Mutt V (1980) Isolation of two novel candidate hormones using a chemical method for finding naturally occurring polypeptides. *Nature* **285:** 417–418.

Tomita T, Kimmel JR, Friesen SR & Mantz FA (1980) Pancreatic polypeptide cell hyperplasia with and without watery diarrhea syndrome. *Journal of Surgical Oncology* **14:** 11–20.

VanDyk C, Inbal A, Kraus L et al (1981) The watery diarrhea syndrome with hypercalcemia—a symptomatic response to phosphate buffer. *Hepate-Gastroenterology* **28:** 58–59.

Verner JV & Morrison AB (1958) Islet cell tumor and a syndrome of refractory watery diarrhea and hypokalemia. *American Journal of Medicine* **25**: 374–380.

Verner JV & Morrison AB (1974) Endocrine pancreatic islet disease with diarrhea. *Annals of Internal Medicine* **133**: 492–500.

Virgolini I, Raderer M, Kurtaran A et al (1994) Vasoactive intestinal peptide-receptor imaging for the localization of intestinal adenocarcinomas and endocrine tumors. *New England Journal of Medicine* **331**: 1116–1121.

Walsh JH & Mayer EA (1993) Gastrointestinal hormones. In Sleisenger MH & Fordtran JS (eds) *Gastrointestinal Disease Pathophysiology/Diagnosis/Management*, pp 18–44. Philadelphia, PA: Saunders.

Watson KJR, Shulkes A, Smallwood RA et al (1985) Watery diarrhea-hypokalemia-achlorhydria syndrome and carcinoma of the esophagus. *Gastroenterology* **88**: 798–803.

Weinstein GS, O'Dorisio TM, Joehl RJ et al (1985) Exacerbation of diarrhea after iodinated contrast agents in a patient with VIPoma. *Digestion Disease Science* **30**: 588–592.

Woltering EA, O'Dorisio TM, Mekhjian HS et al (1986) The response of a non-functional VIP and somatostatin-containing tumour to tolbutamide in vitro. *Scandinavian Journal of Gastroenterology* **21 (supplement)**: 129–135.

Woussen-Colle MC, Gourlet P, Vandermeers A et al (1995) Identification of a new chromogranin B fragment (314-365) in endocrine tumors. *Peptides* **16**: 231–236.

Wu ZC, O'Dorisio TM, Cataland S et al (1979) Effects of pancreatic polypeptide and vasoactive intestinal polypeptide on rat ileal and colonic water and electrolyte transport in vivo. *Digestion Disease Science* **24**: 625–630.

Yagihashi S, Shimoyama N, Morita T et al (1982) Ganglioneuroblastoma containing several kinds of neuronal peptides with watery diarrhea syndrome. *Acta Pathologica Japonica* **32**: 807–814.

Yamaguchi K, Abe K, Adachi I et al (1980) Clinical and hormonal aspects of the watery diarrhea–hypokalemia–achlorhydria (WDHA) syndrome due to vasoactive intestinal polypeptide (VIP)-producing tumor. *Endocrinologia Japonica* **27**: 79–86.

Yamashiro Y, Yamamoto K & Sato M (1982) Loperamide therapy in a child with vipoma-associated diarrhea. *Lancet* **i**: 1413.

Yasunami Y, Funakoshi A, Ryu S et al (1994) In vitro release of vasoactive intestinal polypeptide and pancreatic polypeptide from human VIPoma cells and its inhibition by somatostatin analogue (SMS 201-995). *Surgery* **115**: 713–717.

Yiangou Y, Christofides ND, Blank MA et al (1985) Molecular forms of peptide histidine isoleucine-like immunoreactivity in the gastrointestinal tract. *Gastroenterology* **89**: 516–524.

Yiangou Y, Williams SJ, Bishop AE et al (1987) Peptide histidine–methionine immunoreactivity in plasma and tissue from patients with vasoactive intestinal peptide-secreting tumors and watery diarrhea syndrome. *Journal of Clinical Endocrinology and Metabolism* **64**: 131–139.

7

Glucagonomas

SARAH FRANKTON
STEPHEN R. BLOOM

Glucagonomas are rare α cell tumours of the pancreas which secrete various forms of glucagon and other peptides derived from the pre-pro-glucagon molecule. Although first described in 1942, they have an estimated incidence of only 1 in 20 million; consequently most published reports cite single cases or small numbers grouped with other neuro-endocrine tumours (Bloom and Park, 1987).

In order to clarify the clinical features and therapeutic options in the management of glucagonoma we undertook a retrospective study of 18 patients treated at The Hammersmith Hospital from 1970 to 1995. This is the largest single series to date.

EPIDEMIOLOGY

Glucagonoma may occur sporadically in 80% of cases, the remainder occurring as part of multiple endocrine neoplasia syndrome type 1 (MEN 1). The median age at diagnosis in the former group is 62 years, and it has never been known in children. Patients in the latter group initially present with other features of MEN 1, such as symptoms of primary hyper-parathyroidism, and are screened for neuroendocrine tumours on this basis, or because of a known family history of MEN 1. This group tends to be diagnosed at a younger age, usually below 40 years. There is an approximately equal sex incidence.

An enormous range is seen in the time from first presentation to diagnosis in the sporadic group, ranging from 4 weeks to more than 10 years (median 11 months). Almost half of all cases are referred to a tertiary centre from a dermatologist, and the rest from general physicians, oncologists, general practitioners or gastroenterologists. Around 90% of patients have metastases at presentation, and of these less than 5% have lymph node metastases only. Hepatic metastases are multiple in two-thirds of cases, and usually involve both lobes of the liver. Of the single hepatic metastases, 75% occur in the right lobe. The site of the primary tumour is not always established (27% of cases), although this is becoming less common with

697

Baillière's Clinical Gastroenterology—
Vol. 10, No. 4, December 1996
ISBN 0–7020–2186–5
0950–3528/96/040697 + 9 $12.00/00

the increasing expertise in hepatic angiography. Of these tumours, 17% are found in the head alone, 11% in the head and body, 6% in the body alone and 39% in the tail. This has important implications when planning surgical resection. Tumours in the head may require a Whipple's procedure which is associated with high morbidity and mortality.

CLINICAL FEATURES AND DIAGNOSIS

The most common presenting feature of the glucagonoma syndrome is necrolytic migratory erythema, found in 72% of all patients. The rash usually starts in the groin and perineum and migrates to distal extremities. The initial lesions are erythematous patches, which become raised and may be associated with bullae. These lesions break down and gradually heal, often leading to an area of hyperpigmentation, only to recur in another site. The rash does not only occur in the presence of metastases and is seen in up to 60% of those with benign disease, excluding those with MEN 1 who are asymptomatic and diagnosed on screening.

The cause of this rash is still unknown. A direct effect of glucagon on the skin, prostaglandin release, amino acid or free fatty acid deficiency or zinc deficiency because of the similarity to acrodermatitis enteropathica have all been proposed as the underlying mechanism (Horrobin and Cunnane, 1980; Peterson et al, 1984; Roth et al, 1987). The rash has been reported in a few patients without glucagonoma, who had either coeliac disease or cirrhosis both of which may have been associated with an increase in plasma glucagon or glucagon-like peptides. Patients appear to have normal plasma zinc concentrations, although this is difficult to interpret, since they are usually receiving zinc supplements empirically at the time. Furthermore, plasma and tissue zinc concentrations may not correlate.

Cachexia or marked weight loss occurs in around 67% of all patients, 72% of those with metastases and 40% of those with local disease. This often contributes to death. Diabetes mellitus occurs in around 56% of all cases, only slightly more frequently in those with metastases. This may require insulin therapy. All symptomatic patients appear to suffer from the rash, marked weight loss or diabetes mellitus, or a combination of these.

All mucous membranes may be affected by the rash, leading to angular chelitis (33%), glossitis and stomatitis (33% of all cases). Normochromic normocytic anaemia, occurring in about one-third of cases, is probably due to direct bone marrrow suppression by glucagon. Diarrhoea occurs in about one-fifth of cases, as does psychiatric disturbance. The latter may take the form of clinical depression or paranoid delusions, and seems to occur more frequently in those with metastases. However, the number of patients is small in this category (Prinz et al, 1981; Lambrecht et al, 1987).

The tendency to venous thrombosis is enhanced, occurring in around 11% of all patients, and may be life threatening.

These observations are summarized in Table 1.

Table 1. Clinical features in eighteen patients with proven glucagonoma; malignant and benign disease.

Clinical features	No. of patients $N = 18$	% presenting
Rash	13	72
Metastases at presentation	13	72
Cachexia	12	67
Diabetes	10	56
Angular chelitis	6	33
Anaemia	6	33
Glossitis	5	28
MEN 1	3	17
Diarrhoea	3	17
Psychiatric disturbance	3	17
Zollinger–Ellison syndrome	2	11
Thrombosis	2	11

INVESTIGATION AND DIAGNOSIS

The diagnosis of glucagonoma is made on the basis of a raised fasting plasma glucagon level (>50 pmol/l), together with a demonstrable neuro-endocrine tumour and/or metastatic deposits and characteristic clinical features. Other causes of a raised fasting plasma glucagon level, such as renal or hepatic failure, drugs, prolonged fasting or other stress should be excluded. Plasma glucagon is measured by radioimmunoassay.

Fasting plasma glucagon may only be marginally elevated to 1.5 times the upper limit of normal or be as high as 150 times the upper limit of normal (mean 16 times upper limit of normal). Thus it is important to maintain a high index of suspicion in patients who have other features suggestive of glucagonoma but only marginally elevated fasting plasma glucagon (Edney et al, 1990). This particularly applies to those with MEN 1, or who are being followed up after resection or embolization of a tumour.

Approximately one-fifth of glucagonoma patients also have a raised fasting plasma gastrin level, which may be associated with the Zollinger–Ellison syndrome (White et al, 1985). This is found in one-half of patients at the time of initial diagnosis; the rest usually develop a raised plasma gastrin level between 3 and 6 years after diagnosis. Roughly the same proportion of patients have raised fasting plasma pancreatic polypeptide, although this is less clinically important. The fact that secondary endocrine syndromes may develop even many years after initial diagnosis highlights the importance of annual fasting gut hormone screening, on a lifelong basis.

Pre-operative localization of the tumour improves surgical outcome. Highly selective visceral angiogram or contrast-enhanced computerized tomography (CT) are the investigations of choice, and these may detect tumours missed on transabdominal ultrasound scanning (Wawrukiewicz et al, 1982; Hammond et al, 1994). Choice of investigation may depend on local expertise. There have been previous reports that endoscopic ultrasound is significantly more sensitive in localizing pancreatic tumours than angiography (Rosch et al, 1992), but glucagonomas seem to be successfully localized using the two methods of imaging mentioned above. The role of magnetic resonance imaging has not been evaluated, but it may be a useful non-invasive alternative to CT scanning.

THERAPEUTIC OPTIONS IN LOCAL AND METASTATIC DISEASE

General measures

Most patients are treated empirically with zinc supplements (zinc sulphate 220 mg tds). Other measures which have been tried include high protein diets, topical zinc ointment for the rash, and amino acid infusions. There have been mixed reports of the efficacy of such treatments which are also difficult to evaluate since many patients are already receiving several different therapies.

Diabetic patients may require insulin therapy, and cachexic patients will require appropriate nutritional support.

Aspirin therapy has also been advocated, given the increased thrombotic tendency. Those with Zollinger–Ellison syndrome will also need treatment with omeprazole, and those with psychiatric symptoms appropriate drug treatment and/or psychological therapy. Patients should receive prophylaxis before and after splenectomy, according to current guidelines.

Surgery

Benign disease

Surgical excision remains the treatment of choice for patients with local disease. All patients, whether treated by enucleation of the tumour or distal pancreatectomy and splenectomy, according to the site of the tumour, have a good clinical response. Those who are symptomatic initially undergo symptom relief and normalization of plasma glucagon. Asymptomatic MEN 1 patients, detected by screening, are also seen to have normal plasma glucagon levels post-operatively. Patients can be expected to be well at 1 year follow-up, and at least two-thirds to be alive at 5 years.

Metastatic disease

Even in the presence of metastases, patients enjoy symptom relief after local enucleation of their primary tumour, or resection by distal pancreat-ectomy and splenectomy. This may be the case with or without return of fasting plasma glucagon to within normal values. Around 25% of patients may be expected to have recurrent symptoms within 6 months, and about one-half to be alive at 1 year follow-up. However, a few patients with metastases have survived beyond 5 years with surgical resection of the primary tumour alone (Marynick et al, 1980).

REFERENCES

Ajani JA, Carraso CH, Charnsangavej C et al (1988) Islet cell tumours metastatic to the liver. Effective palliation by sequential percutaneous artery embolization. *Annals of Internal Medicine* **108**: 340–344.

Anderson JV & Bloom SR (1986) Neuroendocrine tumours of the gut: long term therapy with the somatostatin analogue SMS 201-995. *Scandinavian Journal of Gastroenterology* **119 (supplement)**: 115–128.

Arwick AE, Peetz M & Fletchter WS (1981) Dimethyltriazenoimidazole carboxamide therapy of islet cell carcinoma of the pancreas. *Journal of Surgical Oncology* **17**: 321–326.

Bloom SR & Polak JM (1987) Glucagonoma syndrome. *American Journal of Medicine* **82**: 25–36.

Edney JA, Hofmann S, Thompson JS & Kessinger A (1990) Glucagonoma syndrome is an under-diagnosed clinical entity. *American Journal of Surgery* **160**: 625–628 (discussion 628–629).

Hammond PJ, Jackson JA & Bloom SR (1994) Localization of pancreatic endocrine tumours. *Clinical Endocrinology* **40**: 3–14.

Horrobin DF & Cunnane SC (1980) Interactions between zinc, essential fatty acids and prosta-glandins; relevance to acrodermatitis enteropathica, total parenteral nutrition, the glucagonoma syndrome, diabetes, anorexia nervosa and sickle cell anaemia. *Medical Hypothesis* **6**: 277–293.

Jockenhovel F, Lederbogen S, Olbricht T et al (1994) The long acting somatostatin analogue octreotide alleviates symptoms by reducing post-translational conversion of prepro glucagon to glucagon in a patient with malignant glucagonoma, but does not prevent tumor growth. *Clinical Investigation* **72**: 127–133.

Lambrecht ER, van der Loos TL & van der Eerden AH (1987) Retrobulbar neuritis as the first sign of the glucagonoma syndrome. *International Ophthalmology* **11**: 13–15.

Machina T, Marais R & Levin SR (1980) Inhibition of glucagon secretion by diphenylhydantoin in a patient with glucagonoma. *Western Journal of Medicine* **132**: 357–360.

Marynick SP, Fagadau WR & Duncan LA (1980) Malignant glucagonoma syndrome. Response to chemotherapy. *Annals of Internal Medicine* **93**: 453–454.

Peterson LL, Shaw JC, Acott KM et al (1984) Glucagonoma syndrome; in vitro evidence that glucagon increases epidermal arachidonic acid. *Journal of American Academic Dermatology* **11**: 468–473.

Prinz RA, Dorsch TR & Lawrence AM (1981) Clinical aspects of glucagon producing islet cell tumours. *American Journal of Gastroenterology* **76**: 125–131.

Rosch T, Lightdale CJ, Botet JF et al (1992) Localization of pancreatic endocrine tumors by endo-scopic ultrasonography. *New England Journal of Medicine* **326**: 1721–1726.

Roth E, Muhlbacher F, Karner J et al (1987) Free amino acid levels in muscle and liver of a patient with glucagonoma syndrome. *Metabolism* **36**: 7–13.

Schmid R, Allescher HD, Schepp W et al (1988) Effect of somatostatin in skin lesions and concentrations of plasma amino acids in a patient with glucagonoma syndrome. *Hepato-gastroenterology* **35**: 34–37.

Wawrukiewicz AS, Rosch J, Veller FS & Lieberman DA (1982) Glucagonoma and its angiographic diagnosis. *Cardiovascular Interventional Radiology* **5**: 318–324.

White A, Tan K, Gray C et al (1985) Multiple hormone secretion by a human pancreatic glucagonoma in culture. *Regulatory Peptides* **11**: 335–345.

Williams G, Anderson JV, Williams SJ & Bloom SR (1987) Clinical evaluation of SMS 201-995. Long term treatment in gut neuroendocrine tumours, efficacy of oral administration and possible use in non humoral inappropriate TSH hypersecretion. *Acta Endocrinologica* **286 (supplement)**: 26–36.

8

Surgical management of gastrointestinal endocrine tumours

ANTHONY P. GOLDSTONE
DAVID M. SCOTT-COOMBES
JOHN A. LYNN

Arising from the richest source of regulatory peptides outside the brain, the pancreatic islet cell and gut carcinoid tumours produce a variety of 'functioning' endocrine syndromes, or may be hormonally silent or 'non-functioning' (Gilbey et al, 1994; McDermott et al, 1994). A wide spectrum of patients with endocrine gastroenteropancreatic (GEP) tumours are now considered for surgery, whether for curative primary resection or palliative and occasionally curative surgery for metastatic disease (Aldridge and Williamson, 1993; Galland, 1993; Bieligk and Jaffe, 1995; Zogakis and Norton, 1995). Close co-operation between surgeon, endocrinologist, gastroenterologist, anaesthetist, radiologist, pathologist and geneticist is mandatory to ensure a clear plan of action. The rarity and varied natural history of these fascinating tumours makes it difficult to assess appropriate surgical management through prospective randomized clinical trials (Carty et al, 1992; MacFarlane et al, 1995). Experience of the complex management problems is limited, so patients should ideally be managed within tertiary centres. Important lessons can be learnt, however, from retrospective reviews and case reports (Debas and Mulvihill, 1994). Care must be taken if applying findings when different hormone-secreting tumours are reviewed together as one group. Recent advances in our understanding of the genetic (Bale, 1994) and pathological (Capella et al, 1994) processes, parallel medical management (Oberg, 1994), novel methods of pre- and intra-operative localization (Hammond et al, 1994b), intensive care after major gastrointestinal and hepatic surgery, and hepatic transplantation (Anthuber et al, 1996) have influenced the current surgical management of gastrointestinal endocrine tumours.

GENERAL SURGICAL PRINCIPLES

Obsessive pre-operative evaluation gives the patient the optimal chance for a safe peri-operative passage. This includes details of the endocrine

Baillière's Clinical Gastroenterology—
Vol. 10, No. 4, December 1996
ISBN 0–7020–2186–5
0950–3528/96/040707 + 30 $12.00/00

anomaly, accurate localization of the tumour(s), rational appreciation of the need, timing and appropriateness of surgical (and medical) intervention, a strategy for rendering the patient 'safe' peri-operatively and a forewarning of the magnitude of surgery (Lynn, 1993). Advances in radioimmunoassay for plasma tumour hormonal markers and immunocytochemistry have allowed earlier detection, more accurate pathological diagnosis and improved follow-up of patients with endocrine tumours (Capella et al, 1994; Stridsberg et al, 1995).

Tumour localization

Localization of primary tumours and metastatic extent guides appropriate surgery. A range of pre-operative imaging techniques are now available, including transabdominal and endoscopic ultrasound scanning (USS), computed tomography (CT), magnetic resonance imaging (MRI), selective mesenteric arteriography, somatostatin receptor scintigraphy (Krenning et al, 1993), transhepatic portal venous sampling (TPVS), selective arterial secretin and calcium stimulation (Doppman et al, 1990, 1995), each with their own exponents, depending on local experience (Hammond et al, 1994b; Rothmund, 1994). The use of intra-operative ultrasound (IOUS) and more recently hand-held γ probes for tumours radiolabelled by somatostatin analogues has improved the detection of occult tumours and metastases (Schirmer et al, 1993; Zeiger et al, 1993). Some authors have questioned the need for extensive pre-operative imaging (Bottger and Junginger, 1993).

Immunization for splenectomy

Pre-operative localization may also predict the need for splenectomy during distal pancreatic resection (Aldridge and Williamson, 1991). Current guidelines recommend the administration of pneumococcal and *Haemophilus* influenza type b vaccine (if not previously immunized) a minimum of 2 weeks before elective splenectomy or less preferably at the earliest possible post-operative opportunity (Working Party of the British Committee for Standards in Haematology Clinical Haematology Task Force, 1996). Meningococcal immunization is only recommended when travel is planned to areas with an increased risk of group A meningococcal infection.

Pre-operative preparation and anaesthesia

Close liaison with endocrinologists and anaesthetists is needed to ensure adequate pre- and peri-operative stabilization of patients undergoing surgery, many of whom will be severely compromised by endocrine syndromes (Philippe, 1992; Owen, 1993). Specific therapies are used for each syndrome (see individual descriptions below). Somatostatin analogues, such as octreotide, have proved of particular use in carcinoid, glucagonoma and VIPoma (Arnold et al, 1994). Patients typically receive large abdominal incisions and adequate post-operative analgesia is essential. There is no evidence to support the routine post-operative use of octreotide to prevent complications related to pancreatic drainage, such as fistulae (Lange et al, 1992).

Plurihormonal tumours

Gastrointestinal endocrine tumours may display a spectrum of hormone production, from positive immunostaining to raised plasma levels to clinical syndrome from hormone excess. Multiple hormone production is a notorious complicating factor that alters the surgical management of pancreatic endocrine tumours, particularly in multiple endocrine neoplasia type 1 (MEN 1), where multicentric tumours are usual (Mignon et al, 1993). Lifelong follow-up of patients after surgery is essential. In the Hammersmith review, potentially fatal, secondary hormonal syndromes (particularly gastrinoma) occurred in 7% of 353 cases from 7 to 120 months after the diagnosis of the first syndrome (Wynick et al, 1988).

ROLE OF SURGERY IN METASTATIC DISEASE

Surgery is the only available method of cure, in both benign and malignant disease. Abdominal lymphadenopathy is frequently resectable but the benefits of major hepatic surgery must be weighed against the associated morbidity (predominantly sepsis from intra-abdominal collections) and mortality (<5%).

Some studies have shown cure and improved overall survival after surgery for limited, but not extensive (for example, invasion of extra-pancreatic viscera or bulky hepatic metastases) metastatic pancreatic endocrine tumours (Carty et al, 1992) and carcinoids (McEntee et al, 1990; Søreide et al, 1992). Reported 4- to 5-year survival rates were 25–50% in unresected, 48–70% in partially resected and 80–100% in totally resected cases (Zogakis and Norton, 1995). However, less than 10% of cases with neuroendocrine hepatic metastases have localized enough disease to allow complete resection (Ihse et al, 1995). Five-year survival rates of 50–65% have been reported using combination octreotide, streptozotocin–5-fluorouracil (5-FU) cytotoxic and α-interferon therapy (Eriksson and Oberg, 1993). However, all these studies are non-randomized with varying case mixes.

Debulking surgery may palliate symptoms and improve quality of life by reducing hormonal secretion, although duration of symptom relief is variable from 6 to 40 months (Ihse et al, 1995). Delaying the commencement of other therapies may be of long-term benefit (McEntee et al, 1990), as resistance to their action may develop, such as with somatostatin analogues (Wynick et al, 1989), and chemotherapy has associated side-effects (Oberg, 1994). Although outside the remit of this chapter the surgical management of metastatic disease cannot be divorced from the ever-changing medical options (Oberg, 1994). There is some evidence for an antiproliferative benefit of somatostatin analogues in metastatic endocrine GEP tumours (Arnold et al, 1996), in addition to the known benefits in controlling hormone secretion (Arnold et al, 1994; Lamberts et al, 1996). The identification of varying somatostatin receptor subtypes (Kubota et al, 1994; Patel et al, 1995), the presence of receptors for other growth factors (Chaudhry et al, 1993), including VIP (Virgolini et al, 1994), and an improved understanding of tumour genetics (Bale, 1994) may also lead to new therapies for malignant disease.

At the Hammersmith Hospital, we have found that sequential selective hepatic artery embolization provides excellent symptomatic relief in symptomatic metastatic GEP tumours by reducing hormone secretion (Ajani et al, 1988; Gilbey et al, 1994). A variety of different techniques can be used, including stainless steel coils, gelatin sponges, polyvinyl alcohol foam, cyanoacrylate–ethiodized oil mixture and implantable inflatable occluders (Marlink et al, 1990; Ihse et al, 1995; Winkelbauer et al, 1995). Portal vein thrombosis and significant hepatic dysfunction is, however, a contraindication. Acute tumour lysis needs appropriate cover, including octreotide and broad spectrum antibiotics, and careful fluid balance is essential to avoid renal failure from volume depletion, release of vasoactive peptides and contrast load (Gilbey et al, 1994). A post-procedure febrile illness with abnormal liver function is a common occurrence, with associated nausea, vomiting and abdominal pain for up to 10 days. Infection must be continually excluded and the possibility of inadvertent pancreatic or gall-bladder infarction considered.

Response rates of 60% are reported with embolizations repeated every 1–8 months (Ajani et al, 1988). Chemoembolization using doxorubicin and occluding agents has achieved 79% response rates with a mean duration of 9 months and fewer side-effects than occlusion alone (Perry et al, 1994). Improved response rates (80% versus 60%) and mean duration (18 versus 4 months) in metastatic carcinoids have been achieved by combining hepatic artery occlusion with systemic chemotherapy, with similar results in pancreatic tumours (Moertel et al, 1994).

HEPATIC TRANSPLANTATION

Although hepatic transplantation is not usually indicated for secondary malignancy owing to the rapid recurrence with immunosuppression, neuro-endocrine tumours may be an exception as they grow very slowly and metastases are often confined to the liver. Curtiss et al (1995) propose that hepatic transplantation should be considered for patients in whom tumour has either progressed or symptoms of hormone production and mass effect persist despite chemotherapy and embolization. Extrahepatic tumour spread and primary tumour recurrence must be excluded prior to trans-plantation, possibly using somatostatin receptor scintigraphy (Krenning et al, 1993). Transplantation is reserved for a very select few (Anthuber et al, 1996), but in practice is limited by the availability of donor organs. Starzl's group have transplanted five patients with neuroendocrine hepatic metastases (Makowka et al, 1989). The primary pancreatic tumour was also resected at the time of transplantation in three patients. Three patients remain alive at 34, 16 and 7 month follow-up. In another series of 12 patients with neuroendocrine tumour, one-half were alive with a mean survival of 20 months (Schweizer et al, 1993). Tumour recurrence was the cause of death in two patients. However, a recent review reveals that, of 26 patients undergoing transplantation for gut neuroendocrine tumours, only 11 patients (38%) survived beyond 12 months (Frilling et al, 1994). Recent success with cluster transplantation (composite graft of donor liver, stomach, duodenum, pancreas and part of the midgut) for metastatic endocrine tumours (3 year survival of 64% in 14 patients) needs further evaluation (Alessiani et al, 1995).

GASTROINTESTINAL CARCINOID TUMOURS

Carcinoid tumours arise from the enterochromaffin cells (ECL) located throughout the body but primarily within the submucosa of the intestine (85%) and the main bronchi (10%) (Marshall and Bodnarchuk, 1993). Although uncommonly encountered clinically, carcinoid tumours are present in 1% of post-mortem examinations and are the commonest neuro-endocrine tumour of the gastrointestinal tract.

Clinical features and diagnosis

Carcinoid tumours are classified according to their embryological site of ori-gin. The distribution of primary gut carcinoid tumours is shown in Table 1.

Table 1. Distribution of primary gastrointestinal carcinoid tumours.

		Goodwin (1975) (N = 1867)	McDermott et al (1994) (N = 188)
Foregut	Stomach	2%	3.5%
	Duodenum	2%	
Midgut	Small intestine	20%	22%
	Appendix	40%	18%
	Right colon	6%	12%
Hindgut	Rectum	16%	17%

They are often clinically silent (50%) and discovered incidentally at laparotomy or endoscopy as yellow submocosal nodules (Rothmund and Kisker, 1994). Hepatic involvement occurs late after nodal spread, and metastases may also be found in lung and bone.

Small bowel

Carcinoid tumours are the commonest small bowel neoplasm and are often multiple (30%) (McDermott et al, 1994). Two-thirds of patients have metastases and one-third develop the carcinoid syndrome. Of patients with the carcinoid syndrome, 93% have a primary tumour of mid-gut origin.

Small bowel tumours are often symptomatic from bowel obstruction (usually a consequence of a desmoplastic reaction within the small bowel mesentery), carcinoid syndrome, gastrointestinal bleeding, diarrhoea and weight loss (Rothmund and Kisker, 1991). Mesenteric ischaemia and/or venous obstruction may also manifest as severe abdominal pain (angina) in association with meals.

Carcinoid syndrome develops when vasoactive substances (including serotonin, bradykinin, tachykinins, substance P, prostaglandins and histamine) bypass hepatic clearance into the systemic circulation, for example, from hepatic metastases. Typical symptoms are cutaneous flushing (49–90%), diarrhoea (83%), right heart disease (<40%) and broncho-spasm (10%).

Appendix and colorectal

The vast majority of appendiceal carcinoids are incidental and typically patients undergo surgery for 'appendicitis'. In contrast to adenocarcinoma of the colon, carcinoid tumours have a predilection for the right side of the colon (60%) compared with only 13% in the sigmoid colon (Ballantyne et al, 1992). Half of all patients with colonic carcinoids have metastases compared with 80% in colonic adenocarcinoma. The commonest symptoms are abdominal pain and weight loss (Rothmund and Kisker, 1994). Half of all carcinoids of the rectum are asymptomatic and small (<1.0 cm). The more frequent symptoms are bleeding, constipation and rectal pain (Jetmore et al, 1992).

Stomach

Gastric carcinoid tumours were traditionally regarded as rare entities representing less than 3% of all tumours. Recent reports suggest that they are increasingly seen, particularly in association with hypergastrinaemia (Gilligan et al, 1995). Three types of gastric carcinoids are now recognized (Ahlman et al, 1994):

- type I (65%) tumours are associated with hypergastrinaemia from chronic atrophic gastritis and are located in the body and fundus;
- type II (14%) tumours are associated with Zollinger–Ellison syndrome (ZES) in MEN 1;
- type III (21%) are sporadic lesions not associated with elevated gastrin, with 40% located in the antropyloric region.

Between 40% and 50% of lesions associated with hypergastrinaemia are multiple with a low incidence of nodal (16%) and hepatic (4%) metastases, and the 5-year survival is rarely affected. By contrast, sporadic gastric carcinoids display aggressive behaviour and metastasize to lymph nodes and liver (55%).

85–90% are <2 cm in diameter (Rothmund et al, 1990; Geoghegan et al, 1994), <10% are multiple and 10% MEN 1 associated. Although in debate (van Heerden et al, 1992; Bottger and Junginger, 1993), pre-operative localization allows appropriate patient consent (for example risk of diabetes and pancreatic insufficiency), surgical planning (for example Whipple's procedure) and estimation of the number of tumours (especially in MEN 1) and rules out the presence of metastases. CT and USS detect around 30% of tumours (Hammond et al, 1994b). False positives are seen in 9–38% of cases (Pedrazzoli et al, 1994). MRI offers no extra benefit. Angiography remains the gold standard with detection rates of around 60% (Rothmund et al, 1990). In our institution, however, using experienced angiographers, subtraction imaging and superselective catheterization of coeliac and superior mesenteric branches, over 90% may be identified (Geoghegan et al, 1994). This is particularly important in the case of multiple tumours. Percutaneous venous sampling localizes 80–100% but is invasive and expensive and has significant associated complications (Hammond et al, 1994b), while endoscopic USS has its proponents (Thompson et al, 1994). Recently Doppman and our group have found selective intra-arterial calcium stimulation to be the most accurate method of regional pancreatic localization, which is easily performed at the same time as selective angiography (Doppman et al, 1995; O'Shea et al, 1996b).

Intra-operative palpation remains a sensitive procedure (83–95%). IOUS in experienced hands improves detection rates to 89–100%, and also facilitates safe enucleation and avoidance of ductal injury (van Heerden et al, 1992; Zeiger et al, 1993). However, 5–17% of tumours are not found at surgery (Norton et al, 1990; van Heerden et al, 1992; Pedrazzoli et al, 1994), although the use of the newer pre-operative techniques may allow targeted pancreatic resection (Doppman et al, 1995).

Pre-operative preparation and anaesthesia

Diazoxide can be used pre-operatively over several weeks to reduce insulin secretion while surgery is planned (Goode et al, 1986). In the immediate pre-operative period patients receive an intravenous dextrose and potassium infusion. Frequent monitoring of plasma glucose and potassium is needed peri-operatively with 50% dextrose available, particularly during tumour handling. Post-operatively there is typically rebound hyperglycaemia, although this is an unreliable indicator of completeness of tumour resection. Care must be taken to avoid profound hyperglycaemia and water overload–hyponatraemia from dextrose infusions. Octreotide is potentially dangerous in pre-operative stabilization of insulinoma as it may reduce counterregulatory glucagon secretion (Gama et al, 1995).

Surgical strategy for benign insulinoma

Surgical cure is the expected outcome in sporadic insulinoma (Grama et al, 1992a; Geoghegan et al, 1994; Pedrazzoli et al, 1994). The surgical management of MEN 1-associated insulinoma is discussed separately later.

At laparotomy tumours are distributed equally throughout the pancreas. Results from a large international review of 396 patients with benign insulinoma (Rothmund et al, 1990) demonstrated that the majority of tumours in the head of the pancreas may be simply enucleated (75%). Proximal pancreatoduodenectomy (Whipple's) or distal resection is rarely needed with such tumours (13% and 10% respectively). Tumours in the pancreatic body or tail are removed by distal pancreatic resection (57%) or enucleation (41%). Splenectomy can often be avoided if distal pancreatectomy is needed (Aldridge and Williamson, 1991). Complications occurred in 32% of operations, including pancreatic fistula (11%), acute pancreatitis (6%) and intra-abdominal abscess (6%). Thirty-day mortality was only 2%. Complication rates are greater after pancreatic resection than enucleation (Geoghegan et al, 1994). Cure is now achievable in 95% of cases at first operation (Rothmund et al, 1990). Re-operation, usually more extensive surgery for pancreatic head tumours, improved cure rates to 97.5%, but with a higher 30-day mortality of 6%. The presence of multiple tumours was the predominant reason for failure.

Surgical strategy for metastatic insulinoma

Metastatic insulinoma has a poor prognosis with a 50% 5 year survival (Service et al, 1991). Extensive surgery, including hepatic resection, for malignant disease can occasionally allow prolonged disease-free survival for 3–15 years and apparent cure (Grama et al, 1992a; Danforth et al, 1984). Unresectable diseases may be managed with diazoxide, chemotherapy with streptozotocin–5-FU, α-interferon and cautious use of somatostatin analogues to control recurrent hypoglycaemia and to improve prognosis (Eriksson and Oberg, 1993; Oberg, 1994). Sequential hepatic arterial embolization is of symptomatic benefit (Wells et al, 1990) but care must be taken as tumour lysis may acutely aggravate symptoms. Combined with the above strategies, judicious use of debulking surgery can palliate symptoms for many years and delay the need for other therapies (Danforth et al, 1984; Carty et al, 1992; Grama et al, 1992a; Zogakis and Norton, 1995).

Nesidioblastosis and β cell hyperplasia

Nesidioblastosis is a pathological condition of β cell hyperplasia and/or focal adenomatosis, predominantly seen in persistent severe neonatal hyperinsulinaemic hypoglycaemia (Aynsley-Green et al, 1981). In neonates it is managed by subtotal (95% spleen preserving) or total (duodenum preserving) pancreatic resection to avoid the severe neurological consequences of recurrent neuroglycopenia (Dobroschke et al, 1991). Octreotide may also be of therapeutic benefit (Tauber et al, 1994). Although rare, similar multicentric pathology is found in up to 6% of adults with hyperinsulinaemic hypoglycaemia (Rothmund et al, 1990), and is also found in normoglycaemic subjects and in the presence of distinct adenoma. Routine pre-operative imaging, such as angiography, may not alert the surgeon to the multifocal nature (Geoghegan et al, 1994).

These rare cases may account for some of the apparently occult tumours despite pre- and intra-operative imaging. The diagnosis, however, should be based on histological grounds, and not frozen section. If no tumour is found at laparotomy, a small diagnostic biopsy of the pancreatic tail should be performed and further surgery delayed. In adults there is a similar response of β cell hyperplasia or nesidioblastosis to somatostatin analogues (Mozell et al, 1990) and surgery (Farley et al, 1994) to that in neonates. However, medical therapy should be attempted first, as surgery needs to be extensive, with a high risk of post-operative diabetes.

If normal histology is found a vigorous review of the medical diagnosis should follow (including re-exclusion of factitious hypoglycaemia), before further imaging, including intra-arterial calcium stimulation or TPVS, is performed, perhaps allowing targeted surgery (Pedrazzoli et al, 1994). Blind distal pancreatectomy is no longer warranted for occult tumours. Those rare patients with persistently negative imaging and histology, despite these new techniques, should be managed medically.

GASTRINOMA

Clinical features and diagnosis

The eponymous syndrome (ZES) described by Zollinger and Ellison consists of the triad of severe peptic ulcer disease, gastric acid hyper-secretion and neuroendocrine tumour, due to hypergastrinaemia (Gilbey et al, 1994). Historically, affected patients underwent total gastrectomy to control the severe peptic ulcer disease, but now the hypergastrinaemic effects can be controlled by omeprazole in virtually all patients. Gastrinoma is the second commonest islet cell tumour, but frequently occurs in extrapancreatic, particularly duodenal, sites.

Epigastric pain is the most frequent complaint with duodenal ulceration seen in 90% of patients at presentation. Diarrhoea and weight loss are less common (40%) and dysphagia secondary to oesophagitis affects one-third of patients (Bieligk and Jaffe, 1995). Physicians are alerted to ZES by the atypical nature of the peptic ulcers which may be multiple, in unusual sites and recur despite conventional anti-ulcer medication or acid-lowering surgery. The necessary biochemical criteria for a diagnosis of gastrinoma are

1. elevated fasting concentrations of plasma gastrin (>100 pg/ml), and
2. elevated gastric acid secretion (>15 mmol/hour, or >5 mmol/hour after previous gastric surgery).

Patients must stop omeprazole for 2 weeks and H_2-receptor antagonists for 72 hours prior to the tests. A positive secretin provocation test (gastrin increase >200 pg/ml) may be helpful with equivocal cases or where anti-secretory medication cannot be stopped. Hypercalcaemia and renal failure must be excluded. An elevated plasma GAWK, a chromogranin peptide, is specific for gastrinoma in the presence of hypergastrinaemia and although the test lacks sensitivity is unaffected by acid-reducing medication (O'Shea et al, 1996a).

Tumour localization

Ninety per cent of gastrinomas are located in the pancreatic head or duodenal wall in the gastrinoma triangle. Nearly one-half are located in the duodenum, predominantly in the proximal two parts. A 'lymph node' primary gastrinoma located in the peripancreatic region has been described and resection of these tumours has reportedly resulted in cure (Friesen, 1990). Others postulate that these tumours are secondaries from an occult duodenal wall primary tumour (Norton et al, 1992). Other reported primary sites include liver, stomach, jejunum, mesentery, spleen and ovary (Norton, 1994b).

With the development of immunoassays for gastrin, tumours are diagnosed at an early stage and as many as 50% of tumours cannot be localized prior to surgery, particularly duodenal primaries. The sensitivity for different investigations averages 40% for CT, only 20% for USS and MRI, and between 13% and 68% for angiography (Hammond and Bloom, 1993; Rothmund, 1994). Combined secretin stimulation has increased the sensitivity of selective angiography to 75–100%, detecting tumours as small as 1 mm (Doppman et al, 1990; Imamura et al, 1992). Endoscopic USS is poor at detecting small duodenal gastrinomas, but provides good pancreatic imaging in experienced hands (Thompson et al, 1994). Given the current superiority of intra-operative localization techniques (see below), Rothmund (1994) has argued that pre-operative investigation need only exclude advanced metastatic disease.

Pre-operative preparation and anaesthesia

The hypersecretory effects of gastrin can now be effectively controlled with the proton pump inhibitor omeprazole. The usual dose is 80 mg/day by mouth (range 60–120 mg/day) in two divided doses. In the immediate pre- and post-operative periods, intravenous doses of ranitidine that maintain the acid secretion within safe limits are prescribed (Norton, 1994b). A nasogastric tube should be placed and antacid therapy continued after removal of the tumour because of the hypertrophied acid-producing gastric mucosa (Owen, 1993).

Surgical strategy

Around 50% of pancreatic and 10% of duodenal gastrinomas have hepatic metastases at the time of diagnosis, while up to 70% of duodenal tumours <0.5 cm in diameter have local lymph node disease (Hammond and Bloom, 1993). Most patients die from the tumoral process. At surgery nearly all tumours can be identified and complete surgical resection reduces mortality (Ellison, 1995). Tumour clearance produces immediate complete cure rates between 40% and 90%, but nearly half of these patients develop recurrence after 6 years (Norton et al, 1992). Nevertheless, gastrinomas are slow growing and 5-year and 10-year survival rates of 20–42% and 0–30% have been reported for patients with hepatic metastases compared with 90–100% for those patients with localized disease (Norton, 1994b). Therefore an aggressive policy towards complete resection of local tumours is recommended for cure and all patients with sporadic gastrinoma should undergo laparotomy except those with multiple hepatic metastases. The surgical management of MEN 1-associated gastrinoma is discussed separately below. Adequate medical control of gastric acid secretion has made total gastrectomy virtually obsolete, reserved for a minority of patients either unable to tolerate anti-ulcer medication or who have relapsed on medical treatment.

During laparotomy the pancreas and duodenum are thoroughly mobilized out of the retroperitoneum (Kocher manoeuvre, division of inferior and posterior pancreaticoperitoneal attachments, and possibly mobilization of the spleen) and the pancreas is palpated bimanually. IOUS improves detection of intrapancreatic gastrinomas (95%), but is less helpful in duodenal tumours (Zeiger et al, 1993). All suspicious lymph nodes are sent for frozen section and, if tumour is present, the duodenum should be scrutinized. Recent reports have successfully improved intra-operative localization of primary and secondary tumours using radiolabelled somatostatin analogues and a hand-held γ camera (Woltering et al, 1994).

Surgical strategy for duodenal gastrinoma

Palpation of the duodenum misses small tumours, so the following manoeuvres may be undertaken.

1. Methylene blue injection into the gastroduodenal artery reveals small blue-staining tumours (Norton, 1994b).
2. Intra-operative endoscopic transillumination facilitates accurate placement of the duodenotomy incision.
3. Duodenotomy enables close inspection of the medial wall. The surgeon must be careful to avoid damaging both the common bile duct and main pancreatic duct. Any tumour should be excised with a full-thickness elliptical incision. The duodenotomy is closed transversely.
4. IOUS can be used.
5. Lymph node sampling around the pancreatic head should be undertaken.

In a recent series of 31 duodenal gastrinomas, duodenotomy identified all tumours, whereas the success rates for transillumination, palpation and IOUS were 64%, 61% and 26%, respectively (Sugg et al, 1993).

Surgical strategy for pancreatic gastrinoma

With pancreatic tumours the benefits of tumour clearance must be balanced against the risks of major resection (Ellison, 1995). Whenever feasible, pancreatic head tumours are enucleated as this results in excellent long-term survival and avoids the complications of a pancreatoduodenectomy. Tumours of the body and tail of the pancreas, which convey a worse prognosis, are excised as a distal pancreatectomy plus splenectomy as this safely achieves tumour excision with a clear margin.

Indications for pancreatoduodenectomy include multiple duodenal tumours not amenable to local excision, extension beyond duodenal serosa, involvement of the ampulla of Vater and multiple tumours in the pancreatic head (Orloff and Debas, 1995).

Surgical strategy for metastatic gastrinoma

Many patients with liver secondaries are asymptomatic and maintenance omeprazole can effectively control acid secretion in most cases. The best chemotherapeutic regimens achieve only a 50% response rate (Moertel et al, 1992; Eriksson and Oberg, 1993). Resection of a solitary localized lesion has a beneficial result in terms of prolonged disease-free survival, but most patients ultimately develop recurrent disease (Bieligk and Jaffe, 1995). A selective policy towards favourable tumours that can be safely resected with a clear margin is recommended. Hepatic artery embolization is of benefit in reducing tumour bulk in non-resectable disease (Marlink et al, 1990).

MULTIPLE ENDOCRINE NEOPLASIA TYPE 1

MEN 1 is an autosomal dominant familial cancer syndrome, involving the MEN 1 tumour suppressor gene on chromosome 11q13 (Thakker, 1993). Affected individuals develop primary hyperparathyroidism (>90%), gastroenteropancreatic tumours (60–80%, predominantly insulinomas and gastrinomas), pituitary adenomas (50%) and more rarely adrenal tumours, carcinoids and lipomas (Skøgseid et al, 1994).

Surgical consequences of MEN 1 pathology

The surgical management of MEN 1 gastrointestinal endocrine tumours differs from that of sporadic tumours for several reasons (Vassilopoulou-Sellin and Ajani, 1994).

1. The pathological process in MEN 1 involves small, multicentric tumours throughout potentially all pancreatic regions, and in the case of gastrinomas, the duodenum, associated with endocrine cell hyperplasia and even nesidioblastosis. Cure, if at all achievable, therefore requires more extensive surgery.
2. Although similar rates of malignancy to sporadic disease are seen in MEN 1, tumours may behave less malignantly, although there is evidence that some kindreds may exhibit greater malignant potential (Grama et al, 1992b). The increasing efficacy of medical treatment for

the syndromes of hormonal excess may alter the benefits of conservative medical therapy versus aggressive surgery, although this remains much in debate.

3. With biochemical screening in at-risk individuals, disease may be detected early and at a younger age in asymptomatic individuals.

4. The multiple endocrinopathies of MEN 1 complicate matters and multiple gastrointestinal hormone staining and secretion, synchronous or asynchronous, is common. The importance of correct pre-operative localization of pancreatic lesions is therefore paramount. Parathyroidectomy for hypercalcaemia should be performed prior to surgery for gastrinoma, as the former may aggravate hypergastrinaemia and resolution may alter the need for laparotomy (Norton et al, 1987). Surgery for insulinoma should, however, be performed prior to parathyroid surgery (if hypercalcaemia is not life threatening) owing to the more serious risks from hypoglycaemia.

Of patients with ZES, 20–60%, and 10% with insulinomas, have MEN 1 (Vassilopoulou-Sellin and Ajani, 1994) and ZES may be the presenting feature (Benya et al, 1994). All such patients should therefore be evaluated for MEN 1 and family screening performed as needed. Annual fasting gut hormones should be determined in those with or at risk of MEN 1. Oberg has successfully used an exaggerated pancreatic polypeptide response to a standard meal as a screening test (Skøgseid et al, 1994).

Surgical strategy for MEN 1–insulinoma

Insulinoma occurs in up to 35% of MEN 1 patients (Grama et al, 1992b; O'Riordain et al, 1994). In a series of 19 patients from the Mayo Clinic, one patient had unresectable metastatic disease, and one resectable nodal metastases, who remained well at 3 and 11 years post-operatively, suggesting a less aggressive disease process (O'Riordain et al, 1994). Resectable multiple tumours were found in 89%, the median number of tumours being 6 (range 2–16). Conservative gross tumour resection alone (minimal distal resection or tumour enucleation alone) resulted in a greater rate of disease recurrence (two of five patients) than in those having distal subtotal resection (at least 75% of the pancreas, extending at least to the portal vein) together with enucleation of any tumour in the pancreatic head (one of 12 patients). Only one patient had no tumour in the distal pancreas and of the 17 patients with distal tumour 59% had additional tumours that would necessitate such proximal enucleation in addition to distal subtotal resection. Diabetes occurred in only one case who experienced post-operative pancreatic complications. Such a surgical approach may also be regarded as a prophylactic measure for preventing non-insulinoma pancreatic tumours. Total pancreatectomy leads to unacceptable morbidity and mortality (Thompson et al, 1993). Pre-operative USS, CT and angiography are poor at detecting these multiple tumours, but rule out the presence of hepatic metastases (O'Riordain et al, 1994), although some have advised pre-operative use of TPVS (Sheppard et al, 1989; Mignon et al, 1993). IOUS detects 86% and bimanual palpation 45% of the multiple tumours versus 7–12% by CT and 21–37% by angiography (Skøgseid et al, 1995). Although tumours smaller than 0.3 cm were not detected by IOUS there is evidence that only lesions larger than 0.5 cm lead to hyperinsulin-aemia (Grama et al, 1992b). Calcium stimulation may also help in this regard and confirm whether any functioning insulin-producing tumours are in the pancreatic head. This surgical approach of routine subtotal distal pancreatectomy to the portal vein and enucleation of lesions from the pancreatic head is supported by others (Sheppard et al, 1989; Demeure et al, 1991; Grama et al, 1992b). Maintenance diazoxide and somatostatin analogues may be needed for recurrent disease.

Surgical strategy for MEN 1–gastrinoma

Gastrinomas occur in up to 60% of MEN 1 patients, but the surgical strategy in MEN 1 gastrinoma is more controversial than in insulinoma, in view of the higher rate of malignancy (37–47% at presentation) and associated multicentricity (43–55%). Often 5–20 pancreatic or duodenal gastrinomas are found at surgery (Grama et al, 1992b; Mignon et al, 1993; MacFarlane et al, 1995). Standard pre-operative imaging is poor at detect-ing these lesions (Ruszniewski et al, 1993). Earlier reports failed to take into account the high incidence (18–64%) of synchronous pancreatic and duodenal gastrinomas in MEN 1. Although the Ann Arbor group have achieved biochemical cure in 70% of cases, using pre-operative THVS, extensive distal pancreatectomy, enucleation of the pancreatic head, duodenotomy and regional lymph node excision (Thompson, 1995), their success has not been found by others (Mignon et al, 1993).

The NIH and Swedish groups have found early disease recurrence and subsequent development of distant metastases after extensive surgery and duodenal exploration (Grama et al, 1992b; MacFarlane et al, 1995). Although these studies have been criticized for failure to detect all duodenal gastrinomas, delaying surgery until lesions are too large, insufficient lymph node clearance or too conservative pancreatic surgery, the Paris group have shown no biochemical or survival benefit from wide-spread gastrinoma resection in a large series of 45 patients (Mignon et al, 1993). Although 22 of 36 who had surgery were apparently tumour free post-operatively, only one was biochemically cured at 96 months and seven had developed liver metastases after 6–108 months (median 89 months). Overall 5- and 10-year survival rates were similar to those of sporadic ZES at 67% and 63%. Mortality was from progression of gastrinoma in only two of 10 non-surgery-related deaths. They have advocated a conservative approach using medical therapy.

Surgical strategy for MEN 1–carcinoid

The French group also demonstrated gastric ECL hyperplasia in 92% of 14 MEN 1 patients with ZES, undergoing 6-monthly endoscopy, with invasive carcinoid in 36%. Such tumours are unusual in non-MEN 1 ZES suggesting a permissive role of the genetic MEN 1 trait in the promotion of gastric carcinoid with hypergastrinaemia. Regular screening of oxyntic mucosa has therefore been suggested (Ruszniewski et al, 1993).

GLUCAGONOMA

Clinical features and diagnosis

The glucagonoma syndrome has an estimated incidence of 1 per 20 million per year. Clinical features include the characteristic necrolytic migratory erythema rash (predominantly around the perineum, groin, legs and buttocks), mild diabetes, progressive weight loss, stomatitis and glossitis, mental slowing and depression, gastrointestinal disturbance, normochromic and normocytic anaemia (Hammond et al, 1993). Diagnosis is based on these classical findings together with a raised glucagon level in the absence of other causes of hyperglucagonaemia (renal or hepatic failure, drugs, prolonged fasting).

Tumour localization

Only rare cases of extrapancreatic glucagonomas have been described and most pancreatic tumours are larger than 3 cm at diagnosis, with over 75% in the body and tail. CT, USS and selective angiography are therefore usually sufficient for localization and detection of metastases (Hammond et al, 1993). Somatostatin receptor imaging may help in defining metastatic extent (Hammond et al, 1994a).

Pre-operative preparation and anaesthesia

Operative intervention is complicated by the severe cachexia and amino acid deficiency, poor skin protection against infection, anaemia and increased risk of venous thrombosis in glucagonoma. Nasogastric or parenteral feeding, together with topical and oral zinc supplements, and a course of subcutaneous somatostatin analogue should therefore be given pre-operatively for several weeks if these features are present. Perioperative heparin should be considered.

Surgical strategy for localized glucagonoma

In the Hammersmith series of 18 glucagonomas seen between 1970 and 1995, 72% were metastatic at presentation and two of the five non-metastatic tumours were in patients with MEN 1 (Frankton et al, 1996). Surgical cure by resection is consequently less achievable than with insulinoma (Ihse et al, 1995). However, recurrent disease occurred in only one of these five patients, all of whom had full surgical resection, during follow-up of 1–6 years. Excision of the primary tumour more often involves subtotal or distal pancreatic resection than enucleation (Grama et al, 1992a).

Surgical strategy for metastatic glucagonoma

Some surgeons have performed aggressive resection of hepatic and intra-abdominal metastases with at least initial cure (McEntee et al, 1990; Carty et al, 1992). Resection of the pancreatic primary and local lymph-adenopathy together with hepatic transplantation have recently been used for non-distant metastatic glucagonoma (Anthuber et al, 1996). The role of extensive surgery to alter prognosis is uncertain (Zogakis and Norton, 1995).

However, palliative symptomatic benefit may be gained from debulking surgery of abdominal and hepatic metastases (Bieligk and Jaffe, 1995), although few patients have amenable disease. Surgical cure or hepatic debulking was not attempted in our series, where eight out of 12 had multiple hepatic metastases. However, four of 13 patients with metastatic disease had resection of the primary pancreatic tumour, all with symptomatic improvement and three of these were symptom free at 6 months.

There is little evidence of response to cytotoxic chemotherapy with streptozotocin and 5-FU or doxorubicin (Moertel et al, 1992; Eriksson and Oberg, 1993). Symptomatic relief can be achieved medically to good effect with somatostatin analogues (Arnold et al, 1994; Lamberts et al, 1996). Combination therapy with octreotide and sequential hepatic artery embolization is our preferred treatment for unresectable disease (Freimann and Pazdur, 1990; Hammond et al, 1993). In the Hammersmith series 10 out of 12 hepatic embolizations in eight patients gave a good symptomatic response with 50% remaining symptom free after 6 months. Over a follow-up period of 18 months to 11 years (median 3 years) 54% were symptom free, 15% had uncontrolled symptoms (after 3 and 8 years) and 31% had died from their disease (after 18 months to 5 years).

VIPOMA

Clinical features and diagnosis

The VIPoma syndrome was first described by Priest and Alexander, and Verner and Morrison in patients with islet cell tumours with profuse secretory watery diarrhoea (usually >3 l/day). The causative over-production of vasoactive intestinal peptide (VIP) by these tumours was subsequently shown by Bloom (Gilbey et al, 1994). The estimated incidence is 1 per 10 million per year. A stool volume of <700 ml/day effectively excludes the diagnosis. Other associated features include hypokalaemic acidosis, hypochlorhydria (50%), glucose intolerance (glucagon-like effect of VIP on hepatic gluconeogenesis), hypomagnes-aemia, flushing and risk of death from severe dehydration and electrolyte disturbance (Hammond et al, 1993). Diagnosis is made on the basis of a raised VIP >60 pmol/l together with a raised peptide histidine methionine (PHM), a co-secreted VIP-precursor peptide fragment, which may contribute to the clinical syndrome.

Tumour localization

Ninety per cent of VIPomas are pancreatic and are usually large (>3 cm), solitary and within the tail. The remainder are usually ganglioneuro-blastomas, particularly in children, although VIP-secreting adeno-carcinomas and phaeochromocytomas have been described. CT, ultrasound and angiography are usually sufficient for localization of primary and metastatic deposits (Hammond et al, 1993; Bieligk and Jaffe, 1995).

Pre-operative preparation

Rigorous pre-operative resuscitation with fluids and intravenous potassium is essential. The excellent response to somatostatin analogues in over 90% of cases has allowed very rapid (within 24–48 hours) control of the diarrhoea pre-operatively (Arnold et al, 1994). Central venous monitoring may be needed in an acute situation. Peri-operative antacid therapy is recommended as rebound gastric hypersecretion can occasionally occur post-operatively (Bieligk and Jaffe, 1995).

Surgical strategy

Primary tumour excision should be performed where possible (Grama et al, 1992a). Blind distal or subtotal pancreatic resection may be performed if tumour is not found but palpation of the adrenal glands and sympathetic chain for extrapancreatic disease is essential. Fifty per cent of patients have metastases at presentation. Cure has been achieved by resection of limited malignant disease (Nagorney et al, 1983) and selected patients may benefit from more extensive surgery, including Whipple's procedure and hepatic wedge resection, but information is limited (Debas and Mulvihill, 1994). However, in one series all patients who underwent primary tumour and lymph node excision eventually developed liver metastases 2.5–8 years post-operatively (Grama et al, 1992a).

Although debulking of metastatic disease is helpful for symptom relief (Ihse et al, 1995), the good response rate to chemotherapy with strepto-zotocin and 5-FU–doxorubicin (and from some groups α-interferon) may favour medical therapy rather than surgery for extensive hepatic meta-stases (Eriksson and Oberg, 1993), with somatostatin analogue reserved for later use. Hepatic artery embolization or chemoembolization can also be used (Hammond et al, 1993). Five-year and 10-year survival figures of 88% and 25% have been reported for malignant VIPoma (Grama et al, 1992a).

Surgical strategy for MEN 1–VIPoma

It is important to recognize that the co-existence of VIPoma and gastrinoma may often occur in MEN 1, both of which will contribute to diarrhoea. Appropriate pre-operative localization is therefore essential (Vassilopoulou-Sellin and Ajani, 1994).

SOMATOSTATINOMA

Clinical feature and diagnosis

Somatostatinomas are very rare pancreatic tumours with an estimated annual incidence of 1 in 40 million. They are usually (68%) pancreatic, predominantly in the head and body, and are usually large with a mean diameter of 5 cm at diagnosis (Hammond et al, 1993; Bieligk and Jaffe, 1995). They can also arise in the duodenum (19%), ampulla of Vater (3%) and small bowel (3%), when they tend to be smaller. Extrapancreatic tumours are frequently associated with Von Recklinghausen's disease, together with neurofibromatosis and phaeochromocytoma, and contain psammoma bodies (Mao et al, 1995b). Pancreatic tumours more commonly present with the somatostatinoma syndrome (90%), including mild diabetes mellitus, gallstones, steatorrhoea, post-prandial fullness, weight loss and anaemia (Hammond et al, 1993). Extrapancreatic disease usually presents with pancreatitis, obstructive jaundice, intestinal haemorrhage or obstruction or abdominal pain, rather than symptoms of excess somatostatin secretion (O'Brien et al, 1993). An elevated fasting somatostatin level confirms the diagnosis, although levels are lower in duodenal disease.

Tumour localization

The large size of pancreatic tumours and metastases in over 70% of cases means that USS and CT can detect tumours, perhaps combined with angiography. Duodenal tumours are usually benign and are found during endoscopy or barium studies. However, CT scans should be performed to look for metastatic disease, as tumours larger than 2 cm are usually malignant.

Surgical strategy

Pancreatic tumours can rarely be cured owing to tumour extent, less than 10% in some series, and a Whipple's procedure is usually needed. Debulking surgery is, however, warranted for symptom palliation. Prophylactic cholecystectomy should be considered at the time of laparotomy. Prognosis is variable depending on tumour aggressiveness and stage, ranging from 1 week to 5 years from diagnosis to 25 years from onset of symptoms. Duodenal tumours are more often amenable to curative resection, although Whipple's procedure is often needed. Hepatic embolization can be used for palliation and partial responses have been seen with streptozotocin and 5-FU (Bieligk and Jaffe, 1995).

OTHER HORMONAL SYNDROMES

ACTHomas

Ectopic production of adrenocorticotrophic hormone and corticotropin-releasing hormone by pancreatic islet tumours can produce Cushing's syndrome. In a recent series of 12 patients (Amikura et al, 1995), 83% had liver metastases at diagnosis (usually with concomitant ZES, present in 75%) and none of those who underwent aggressive surgery, including distal pancreatectomy and hepatic resection, had biochemical cure. All the latter patients and 75% in total needed bilateral adrenalectomy to control the Cushing's syndrome. Fifty per cent died of the disease within 2.5 years of diagnosis. Hepatic embolization may help to control tumour bulk symptoms. Somatostatin analogues may also partially control hyper-cortisolism (Lamberts et al, 1994).

PTHrPomas

Rare cases of islet cell tumours associated with hypercalcaemia and ectopic production of parathyroid hormone (PTH)-related protein (PTHrP) have been described (Mao et al, 1995a). PTHrP displays homology to PTH and is able to stimulate osteoclastic bone resorption and renal tubular calcium reabsorption via its receptor. These tumours are extremely vascular and virtually always malignant. Hepatic embolization has been used to control hypercalcaemia (Tarver and Birch, 1992). Somatostatin analogues are extremely successful in reducing PTHrP secretion (Wynick et al, 1990). Despite metastases some patients are alive 8–11 years after diagnosis. One patient at our institution has been cured following excision of the primary tumour and hepatic transplantation.

GHRHomas

Rare ectopic secretion of growth-hormone-releasing hormone can lead to pituitary somatotroph hyperplasia or adenoma and acromegaly. Manage-ment is surgical resection where possible, but hepatic embolization and octreotide have been used to control hormone secretion in unresectable metastatic disease (Hammond et al, 1993).

PPomas and neurotensinomas

Pancreatic polypeptide is secreted by 75% of VIPomas and 50% of glucagonomas, and 10% of VIPomas secrete neurotensin, although immunostaining for these peptides is even more common. No particular hormonal syndrome has been attributed to their secretion and their surgical management is identical to that of the underlying syndrome (Hammond et al, 1993).

NON-FUNCTIONING NEUROENDOCRINE TUMOURS OF THE PANCREAS

Neuroendocrine tumours which lack an associated syndrome owing to the absence of active peptide production are termed non-functioning. Such tumours may be silent either because they produce peptides in insufficient quantities (or not at all) or because the hormones they produce, such as pancreatic polypeptide, do not manifest any specific clinical signs.

Clinical features and diagnosis

Increased plasma concentrations of pancreatic polypeptide are found in 22–77% of functioning tumours and 75% of non-functioning tumours (Hammond et al, 1993). Absence of an endocrine syndrome may explain why patients present later than their functioning counterparts, usually in the presence of metastases, and with a worse prognosis (median survival 40 versus 60 months) (Eriksson and Oberg, 1993). These tumours are slow-growing and most commonly located within the pancreatic head. In the Hammersmith series ($N = 20$), the commonest presenting features were a mass (40%), obstructive jaundice (35%), abdominal pain (35%) and weight loss (30%) (Cheslyn Curtis et al, 1993). Most tumours are diagnosed using CT and angiography. Typical features are a large mass (>5 cm), calcification and pronounced vascularity.

Surgical strategy

Tumour resection is feasible in the majority of patients, but as 80% of these tumours are malignant, curative resection is only possible in 30–50% (Cheslyn Curtis et al, 1993; Bieligk and Jaffe, 1995). Since prolonged survival occurs with advanced disease, it is difficult to determine the benefit of curative resection over palliative treatment. Nevertheless, the agreed treatment of choice is surgical resection (Cheslyn Curtis et al, 1993; Debas and Mulvihill, 1994; Bieligk and Jaffe, 1995) as they respond poorly to chemotherapy (Moertel et al, 1992; Oberg, 1994). There is some evidence emerging for anti-proliferative effects of somatostatin analogues (Arnold et al, 1996). In the Hammersmith series, 14 of 20 patients underwent resection (of whom 10 had apparently total resection) and three surgical bypass. For those patients who underwent curative resection and left hospital alive ($N = 9$), the median survival was 36 months from surgery (range 12–36 months) (Cheslyn Curtis et al, 1993).

SUMMARY

The surgical management of gastrointestinal endocrine tumours must involve a multidisciplinary approach. The importance of accurate diagnosis, rendering the patient safe, and, in our opinion, localizing the tumour(s) before embarking on surgery cannot be overemphasized. Surgery is the only available treatment for cure. Occult primary tumours are now rarely a problem with novel imaging techniques, which can also improve detection and hence clearance of local spread. Surgical management in extensive metastatic or multicentric disease is less rigidly defined, and is dependent on the endocrine syndrome. A better understanding of tumour pathology, for example in MEN 1, has not always simplified matters. An appreciation of the benefits of chemotherapy, use of somatostatin analogues and hepatic artery embolization are vital to target appropriate palliative surgery. Hepatic transplantation may have an increasing role in the future. Surgical strategies must adapt to new medical treatments. If therapeutically relevant, advances in tumour biology (for example somatostatin receptor subtypes and growth factors) will influence surgical strategies in the future.

Acknowledgement

A.P. Goldstone is supported by the UK Medical Research Council.

REFERENCES

Ahlman H, Wangberg B, Tisell LE et al (1994) Clinical efficacy of octreotide scintigraphy patients with midgut carcinoid tumours and evaluation of intraoperative scintillation detection. *British Journal of Surgery* **81:** 1144–1149.

Ajani JA, Carrasco CH, Charnsangavej C et al (1988) Islet cell tumors metastatic to the liver: effective palliation by sequential hepatic artery embolization. *Annals of Internal Medicine* **108:** 340–344.

Akerstrom G, Makridis C & Johansson H (1991) Abdominal surgery in patients with midgut carcinoid tumors. *Acta Oncologica* **30:** 547–553.

Aldridge MC & Williamson RCN (1991) Distal pancreatectomy with and without splenectomy. *British Journal of Surgery* **78:** 976–979.

Aldridge MC & Williamson RCN (1993) Surgery of endocrine tumours of the pancreas. In Lynn JA & Bloom SR (eds) *Surgical Endocrinology*, pp503–520. Oxford: Butterworth Heinemann.

Alessiani M, Tzakis A, Todo S et al (1995) Assessment of five-year experience with abdominal organ cluster transplantation. *Journal of the American College of Surgeons* **180:** 1–9.

Amikura K, Alexander HR, Norton JA et al (1995) Role of surgery in management of adrenocorticotropic hormone-producing islet cell tumours of the pancreas. *Surgery* **118:** 1125–1130.

Anthuber M, Jauch KW, Briegel J et al (1996) Results of liver transplantation for gastroenteropancreatic tumor metastases. *World Journal of Surgery* **20:** 73–76.

Arnold R, Frank M & Kajdan U (1994) Management of gastroenteropancreatic endocrine tumors: the place of somatostatin analogues. *Digestion* **55 (supplement 3):** 107–113.

Arnold R, Trautmann ME, Creutzfeldt W et al (1996) Somatostatin analogue octreotide and inhibition of tumour growth in metastatic endocrine gastroenteropancreatic tumours. *Gut* **38:** 430–438.

Aynsley-Green A, Polak JM, Bloom SR et al (1981) Nesidioblastosis of the pancreas: Defition of the syndrome and the management of the severe neonatal hyperinsulinaemic hypoglycaemia. *Archives of Disease in Childhood* **56:** 496–508.

Bale AE (1994) Molecular mechanisms of neoplasia in multiple endocrine neoplasia type l-related and sporadic tumors of the pancreatic islet cells. *Endocrinological and Metabolic Clinics of North America* **23:** 109–115.

Ballantyne GH, Savoca PE, Flannery JT et al (1992) Incidence and mortality of carcinoids of the colon. Data from the Connecticut Tumor Registry. *Cancer* **69:** 2400–2405.

Benya RV, Metz DC, Venzon DJ et al (1994) Zollinger–Ellison syndrome can be the initial endocrine manifestation in patients with multiple endocrine neoplasia-type I. *American Journal of Medicine* **97:** 436–444.

Bieligk S & Jaffe BM (1995) Islet cell tumors of the pancreas. *Surgical Clinics of North America* **75:** 1025–1040.

Bottger TC & Junginger T (1993) Is preoperative radiographic localization of islet cell tumors in patients with insulinoma necessary? *World Journal of Surgery* **17:** 427–432.

Burke AP, Sobin LH, Federspiel BH et al (1990) Carcinoid tumors of the duodenum. A clinicopathologic study of 99 cases. *Archives of Pathology and Laboratory Medicine* **114:** 700–704.

Capella C, Heitz PU, Hofler H et al (1994) Revised classification of neuroendocrine tumors of the lung, pancreas and get. *Digestion* **55 (supplement 3):** 11–23.

Carty SE, Jensen RT & Norton JA (1992) Prospective study of aggressive resection of metastatic pancreatic endocrine tumors. *Surgery* **112:** 1024–1032.

Chaudhry A, Funa K & Oberg K (1993) Expression of growth factor peptides and their receptors in neuroendocrine tumors of the digestive system. *Acta Oncologica* **32:** 107–114.

Cheslyn Curtis S, Sitaram V & Williamson RC (1993) Management of non-functioning neuro-endocrine tumours of the pancreas. *British Journal of Surgery* **80:** 625–627.

Curtiss SI, Mor E, Schwartz ME et al (1995) A rational approach to the use of hepatic transplantation in the treatment of metastatic neuroendocrine tumors. *Journal of the American College of Surgeons* **180:** 184–187.

Danforth DN, Gorden P & Brennan MF (1984) Metastatic insulin-secreting carcinoma of the pancreas: clinical course and the role of surgery. *Surgery* **96:** 1027–1037.

Davies MG, O'Dowd G, McEntee GP & Hennessy TP (1990) Primary gastric carcinoids: a view on management. *British Journal of Surgery* **77:** 1013–1014.

Debas HT & Mulvihill SJ (1994) Neuroendocrine gut neoplasms. Important lessons from uncommon tumors. *Archives of Surgery* **129:** 965–971.

Demeure MJ, Klonoff DC, Karam JH et al (1991) Insulinomas associated with multiple endocrine neoplasia type I: the need for a different surgical approach. *Surgery* **110:** 998–1004.

Dobroschke J, Linder R & Otten A (1991) Surgical treatment of nesidioblastosis in childhood. *Progress in Pediatric Surgery* **26:** 84–91.

Doppman JL, Miller DL, Chang R et al (1990) Gastrinomas: localization by means of selective intra-arterial injection of secretin. *Radiology* **174:** 25–29.

Doppman JL, Chang R, Fraker DL et al (1995) Localization of insulinomas to regions of the pancreas by intra-arterial stimulation with calcium. *Annals of Internal Medicine* **123:** 269–273.

Ellison EC (1995) Forty-year appraisal of gastrinoma. Back to the future. *Annals of Surgery* **222:** 511–521.

Erikson B & Oberg K (1993) An update of the medical treatment of malignant endocrine pancreatic tumors. *Acta Oncologica* **32:** 203–208.

Farley DR, van Heerden JA & Myers JL (1994) Adult pancreatic nesidioblastosis. Unusual presenta-tions of a rare entity. *Archives of Surgery* **129:** 329–332.

Frankton S, Goldstone AP, Wilding JPH & Bloom SR (1996) Long-term follow up of eighteen glucagonomas. *Journal of Endocrinology* **148 (supplement):** P371.

Freimann J & Pazdur R (1990) Hepatic arterial embolization for treatment of glucagonomas: anti-neoplastic and palliative benefits. *American Journal of Clinical Oncology* **13:** 271–275.

Friesen SR (1990) Are 'aberrant nodal gastrinomas' pathogenetically similar to 'lateral aberrant thyroid' nodules? *Surgery* **107:** 236–238.

Frilling A, Rogiers X, Knofel WT & Broelsch CE (1994) Liver transplantation for metastatic carcinoid tumors. *Digestion* **55 (supplement):** 104–106.

Galland RB (1993) Surgical aspects of carcinoid tumours. In Lynn JA & Bloom SR (eds) *Surgical Endocrinology*, pp494–502. Oxford: Butterworth Heinemann.

Gama R, Marks V, Wright J & Teale JD (1995) Octreotide exacerbated fasting hypoglycaemia in a patient with a proinsulinoma: the glucostatic importance of pancreatic glucagon. *Clinical Endocrinology* **43:** 117–120.

Geoghegan JG, Jackson JE, Lewis MP et al (1994) Localization and surgical management of insulinoma. *British Journal of Surgery* **81:** 1025–1028.

Gilbey SG, Turner RC, Wynick D & Bloom SR (1994) Endocrine tumours of the pancreas. In Khan CR & Weir GC (eds) *Diabetes Mellitus*, pp1000–1022. Philadelphia, PA: Lea & Febiger.

Gilligan CJ, Lawton GP, Tang LH et al (1995) Gastric carcinoid tumors: the biology and therapy of an enigmatic and controversial lesion. *American Journal of Gastroenterology* **90:** 338–352.

Goode PN, Farndon JR, Anderson J et al (1986) Diazoxide in the management of patients with insulinoma. *World Journal of Surgery* **10:** 586–592.

Goodwin JD (1975) Carcinoid tumors. An analysis of 2837 cases. *Cancer* **36:** 560–569.

Grama D, Eriksson B, Martensson H et al (1992a) Clinical characteristics, treatment and survival in patients with pancreatic tumors causing hormonal syndromes. *World Journal of Surgery* **16:** 632–639.

Grama D, Skøgseid B, Wilander E et al (1992b) Pancreatic tumors in multiple endocrine neoplasia type 1: clinical presentation and surgical treatment. *World Journal of Surgery* **16:** 611–618.

Hammond PJ & Bloom SR (1993) Searching for gastrinomas. *British Medical Journal* **307:** 4–5.

Hammond PJ, Gilbey SG, Wynick D & Bloom SR (1993) Glucagonoma, VIPoma, somatostatinoma, other hormones, and nonfunctional tumors. In Mazzaferri EL & Samaan NA (eds) *Endocrine Tumors*, pp457–483. Oxford: Blackwell Scientific Publications.

Hammond PJ, Arka A, Peters AM et al (1994a) Localization of metastatic gastroenteropancreatic tumours by somatostatin receptor scintigraphy with [¹¹¹In-DTPA-D-Phel]-octreotide. *Quarterly Journal of Medicine* **87**: 83–88.

Hammond PJ, Jackson JA & Bloom SR (1994b) Localization of pancreatic endocrine tumours. *Clinical Endocrinology* **40**: 3–14.

Ihse I, Persson B & Tibblin S (1995) Neuroendocrine metastases of the liver. *World Journal of Surgery* **19**: 76–82.

Imamura M, Kanda M, Takahashi K et al (1992) Clinicopathological characteristics of duodenal microgastrinomas. *World Journal of Surgery* **16**: 703–710.

Jetmore AB, Ray JE, Gathright JB Jr et al (1992) Rectal carcinoids: the most frequent carcinoid tumor. *Diseases of the Colon and Rectum* **35**: 717–725.

Krenning EP, Kwekkeboom DJ, Bakker WH et al (1993) Somatostatin receptor scintigraphy with [¹¹¹In-DTPA-D-Phel]- and [¹²³I-Tyr3]-octreotide: the Rotterdam experience with more than 1000 patients. *European Journal of Nuclear Medicine* **20**: 716–731.

Kubota A, Yamada Y, Kagimoto S et al (1994) Identification of somatostatin receptor subtypes and an implication for the efficacy of somatostatin analogue SMS 201-995 in treatment of human endocrine tumors. *Journal of Clinical Investigation* **93**: 1321–1325.

Lamberts SW, de Herder WW, Krenning EP & Reubi JC (1994) A role of (labeled) somatostatin analogs in the differential diagnosis and treatment of Cushing's syndrome. *Journal of Clinical Endocrinology and Metabolism* **78**: 17–19.

Lamberts SWJ, Van der Lely A-J, de Herder WW & Hofland LJ (1996) Drug therapy: octreotide. *New England Journal of Medicine* **334**: 246–254.

Lange JR, Steinberg SM, Doherty GM et al (1992) A randomized, prospective trial of postoperative somatostatin analogue in patients with neuroendocrine tumors of the pancreas. *Surgery* **112**: 1033–1037.

Lynn JA (1993) The principles of endocrine surgery. In Lynn JA & Bloom SR (eds) *Surgical Endocrinology*, pp 1–4. Oxford: Butterworth Heinemann.

MacFarlane MP, Fraker DL, Alexander R et al (1995) Prospective study of surgical resection of duodenal and pancreatic gastrinomas in multiple endocrine neoplasia type 1. *Surgery* **118**: 973–980.

MacGillivray DC, Synder DA, Drucker W & ReMine SG (1991) Carcinoid tumors: the relationship between clinical presentation and the extent of disease. *Surgery* **110**: 68–72.

Makowka L, Tzakis AG, Mazzaferro V et al (1989) Transplantation of the liver for metastatic endocrine tumors of the intestine and pancreas. *Surgery, Gynecology and Obstetrics* **168**: 107–111.

Mao C, Carter P, Schaefer P et al (1995a) Malignant islet cell tumor associated with hypercalcemia. *Surgery* **117**: 37–40.

Mao C, Shah A, Hanson DJ & Howard JM (1995b) Von Recklinghausen's disease associated with duodenal somatostatinoma: contrast of duodenal versus pancreatic somatostatinomas. *Journal of Surgical Oncology* **59**: 67–73.

Marlink RG, Lokich JJ, Robins JR & Clouse ME (1990) Hepatic arterial embolization for metastatic hormone-secreting tumors. Technique, effectiveness, and complications. *Cancer* **65**: 2227–2232.

Marshall JB & Bodnarchuk G (1993) Carcinoid tumors of the gut. Our experience over three decades and review of the literature. *Journal of Clinical Gastroenterology* **16**: 123–129.

McDermott EW, Guduric B & Brennan MF (1994) Prognostic variables in patients with gastrointestinal carcinoid tumours. *British Journal of Surgery* **81**: 1007–1009.

McEntee GP, Nagorney DM, Kvols LK et al (1990) Cytoreductive hepatic surgery for neuroendocrine tumors. *Surgery* **108**: 1091–1096.

Mignon M, Ruszniewski P, Podevin P et al (1993) Current approach to the management of gastrinoma and insulinoma in adults with multiple endocrine neoplasia type I. *World Journal of Surgery* **17**: 489–497.

Modlin IM, Lawton GP, Miu K et al (1996) Pathophysiology of the fundic enterochromaffin-like (ECL) cell and gastric carcinoid tumours. *Annals of the Royal College of Surgeons of England* **78**: 133–138.

Moertel CG, Weiland LH, Nagorney DM & Dockerty MB (1987) Carcinoid tumor of the appendix: treatment and prognosis. *New England Journal of Medicine* **317**: 1699–1701.

Moertel CG, Lefkopoulo M, Lipsitz S et al (1992) Streptozocin–doxorubicin, streptozocin–fluorouracil or chlorozotocin in the treatment of advanced islet-cell carcinoma. *New England Journal of Medicine* **326:** 519–523.

Moertel CG, Johnson CM, McKusick MA et al (1994) The management of patients with advanced carcinoid tumors and islet cell carcinomas. *Annals of Internal Medicine* **120:** 302–309.

Mozell EJ, Woltering EA, O'Dorisio TM et al (1990) Adult onset nesidioblastosis: response of glucose, insulin, and secondary peptides to therapy with Sandostatin. *American Journal of Gastroenterology* **85:** 181–188.

Nagorney DM, Bloom SR, Polak JM & Blumgart LH (1983) Resolution of recurrent Verner–Morrison syndrome by resection of metastatic VIPoma. *Surgery* **93:** 348–353.

Norton JA (1994a) Neuroendocrine tumors of the pancreas and duodenum. *Current Problems in Surgery* **31:** 77–156.

Norton JA (1994b) Surgical management of carcinoid tumors: role of debulking and surgery for patients with advanced disease. *Digestion* **55 (supplement 3):** 98–103

Norton JA, Cornelius MJ, Doppman JL et al (1987) Effect of parathyroidectomy in patients with hyperparathyroidism, Zollinger–Ellison syndrome, and multiple endocrine neoplasia type I: a prospective study. *Surgery* **102:** 958–966.

Norton JA, Shawker TH, Doppman JL et al (1990) Localization and surgical treatment of occult insulinomas. *Annals of Surgery* **212:** 615–620.

Norton JA, Doppman JL & Jensen RT (1992) Curative resection in Zollinger–Ellison syndrome. Results of a 10-year prospective study. *Annals of Surgery* **215:** 8–18.

O'Brien TD, Chejfec G & Prinz RA (1993) Clinical features of duodenal somatostatinomas. *Surgery* **114:** 1144–1147.

O'Riordain DS, O'Brien T, van Heerden JA et al (1994) Surgical management of insulinoma associated with multiple endocrine neoplasia type I. *World Journal of Surgery* **18:** 488–493.

O'Shea D, Abourawi FI, Williams S & Bloom SR (1996a) Elevated gastrin levels in clinical practice. *Journal of Endocrinology* **148 (supplement):** OC23.

O'Shea D, Rohrer-Theus AW, Lynn JA et al (1996b) Localization of insulinomas by selective intra-arterial calcium injection. *Journal of Clinical Endocrinology and Metabolism* **81:** 1623–1627.

Oberg K (1994) Treatment of neuroendocrine tumors. *Cancer Treatment Reviews* **20:** 331–355.

Orloff SL & Debas HT (1995) Advances in the management of patients with Zollinger–Ellison syndrome. *Surgical Clinics of North America* **75:** 511–524.

Owen R (1993) Anaesthetic considerations in endocrine surgery. In Lynn JA & Bloom SR (eds) *Surgical Endocrinology*, pp 71–84. Oxford: Butterworth Heinemann.

Patel YC, Greenwood MT, Panetta R et al (1995) The somatostatin receptor family. *Life Sciences* **57:** 1249–1265.

Pedrazoli S, Pasquali C & Alfano D-A (1994) Surgical treatment of insulinoma. *British Journal of Surgery* **81:** 672–676.

Perry LJ, Stuart K, Stokes KR & Clouse ME (1994) Hepatic arterial chemoembolization for metastatic neuroendocrine tumors. *Surgery* **116:** 1111–1116.

Philippe J (1992) APUDomas: acute complications and their medical management. In *Baillière's Clinical Endocrinology and Metabolism*, vol. 6, pp 217–228. London: Baillière Tindall.

Rothmund M (1994) Localization of endocrine pancreatic tumours. *British Journal of Surgery* **81:** 164–166.

Rothmund M & Kisker O (1994) Surgical treatment of carcinoid tumors of the small bowel, appendix, colon and rectum. *Digestion* **55 (supplement 3):** 86–91.

Rothmund M, Angelini L, Brunt LM et al (1990) Surgery for benign insulinoma: an international review. *World Journal of Surgery* **14:** 393–398.

Ruszniewski P, Podevin P, Cadiot G et al (1993) Clinical, anatomical, and evolutive features of patients with the Zollinger–Ellison syndrome combined with type I multiple endocrine neoplasia. *Pancreas* **8:** 295–304.

Sauven P, Ridge JA, Quan SH & Sigurdson ER (1990) Anorectal carcinoid tumors. Is aggressive surgery warranted? *Annals of Surgery* **211:** 67–71.

Schirmer WJ, O'Dorisio TM, Schirmer TP et al (1993) Intraoperative localization of neuroendocrine tumors with ^{125}I-TYR(3)-octreotide and a hand-held gamma-detecting probe. *Surgery* **114:** 745–751.

Schweizer RT, Alsina AE, Rosson R & Bartus SA (1993) Liver transplantation for metastatic neuroendocrine tumors. *Transplantation Proceedings* **25:** 1973.

Service FJ (1995) Hypoglycemic disorders. *New England Journal of Medicine* **32:** 1144–1152.

Service FJ, McMahon MM, O'Brien PC & Ballard DJ (1991) Functioning insulinoma—incidence, recurrence, and long-term survival of patients: a 60-year study. *Mayo Clinic Proceedings* **66:** 711–719.

Sheppard BC, Norton JA, Doppman JL et al (1989) Management of islet cell tumors in patients with multiple endocrine neoplasia: a prospective study. *Surgery* **106:** 1108–1117.

Skøgseid B, Rastad J & Oberg K (1994) Multiple endocrine neoplasia type 1. Clinical features and screening. *Endocrinological and Metabolic Clinics of North America* **23:** 1–18.

Skøgseid B, Grama D, Rastad J et al (1995) Operative tumour yield obviates preoperative pancreatic tumour localization in multiple endocrine neoplasia type 1. *Journal of Internal Medicine* **238:** 281–288.

Søreide O, Berstad T, Bakka A et al (1992) Surgical treatment as a principle in patients with advanced abdominal carcinoid tumors. *Surgery* **111:** 48–54.

Stridsberg M, Oberg K, Li Q et al (1995) Measurements of chromogranin A, chromogranin B (secretogranin I), chromogranin C (secretogranin II) and pancreastatin in plasma and urine from patients with carcinoid tumours and endocrine pancreatic tumours. *Journal of Endocrinology* **144:** 49–59.

Sugg SL, Norton JA, Fraker DL et al (1993) A prospective study of intraoperative methods to diagnose and resect duodenal gastrinomas. *Annals of Surgery* **218:** 138–144.

Sugimoto E, Lorelius LE, Eriksson B & Oberg K (1995) Midgut carcinoid tumours. CT appearance. *Acta Radiologica* **36:** 367–371.

Tarver DS & Birch SJ (1992) Case report: life-threatening hypercalcaemia secondary to pancreatic tumour secreting parathyroid hormone-related protein—successful control by hepatic arterial embolization. *Clinical Radiology* **46:** 204–205.

Tauber MT, Harris AG & Rochiccioli P (1994) Clinical use of the long acting somatostatin analogue octreotide in pediatrics. *European Journal of Pediatrics* **153:** 304–310.

Thakker RV (1993) The molecular genetics of the multiple endocrine neoplasia syndromes. *Clinical Endocrinology* **38:** 1–14.

Thirlby RC (1995) Management of patients with gastric carcinoid tumors. *Gastroenterology* **108:** 296–297.

Thompson NW (1995) The surgical management of hyperparathyroidism and endocrine disease of the pancreas in the multiple endocrine neoplasia type 1 patient. *Journal of Internal Medicine* **238:** 269–280.

Thompson GB, Service FJ, van Heerden JA et al (1993) Reoperative insulinomas, 1927 to 1992: an institutional experience. *Surgery* **114:** 1196–1204.

Thompson NW, Czako PF, Fritts LL et al (1994) Role of endoscopic ultrasonography in the localization of insulinomas and gastrinomas. *Surgery* **116:** 1131–1138.

van Heerden JA, Grant CS, Czako PF et al (1992) Occult functioning insulinomas: which localizing studies are indicated? *Surgery* **112:** 1010–1014.

Vassilopoulou-Sellin R & Ajani J (1994) Islet cell tumors of the pancreas. *Endocrinological and Metabolic Clinics of North America* **23:** 53–65.

Veall GR, Peacock JE, Bax ND & Reilly CS (1994) Review of the anaesthetic management of 21 patients undergoing laparotomy for carcinoid syndrome. *British Journal of Anaesthetics* **72:** 335–341.

Virgolini I, Raderer M, Kurtaran A et al (1994) Vasoactive intestinal peptide-receptor imaging for the localization of intestinal adenocarcinomas and endocrine tumors. *New England Journal of Medicine* **331:** 1116–1121.

Wells JL, Heath DA & West RJ (1990) Hepatic artery embolization in the treatment of intractable hypoglycaemia. *Journal of the Royal Society of Medicine* **83:** 592–593.

Winkelbauer FW, Niederle B, Pietschmann F et al (1995) Hepatic artery embolotherapy of hepatic metastases from carcinoid tumors: value of using a mixture of cyanoacrylate and ethiodized oil. *American Journal of Roentgenology* **165:** 323–327.

Woltering EA, Barrie R, O'Dorisio TM et al (1994) Detection of occult gastrinomas with iodine 125-labeled lanreotide and intraoperative gamma detection. *Surgery* **116:** 1139–1146.

Working Party of the British Committee for Standards in Haematology Clinical Haematology Task Force (1996) Guidelines for the prevention and treatment of infection in patients with an absent or dysfunctional spleen. *British Medical Journal* **312:** 430–434.

Wynick D, Williams SJ & Bloom SR (1988) Symptomatic secondary hormone syndromes in patients with established malignant pancreatic endocrine tumors. *New England Journal of Medicine* **319:** 605–607.

Wynick D, Anderson JV, Williams SJ & Bloom SR (1989) Resistance of metastatic pancreatic endocrine tumours after long-term treatment with the somatostatin analogue octreotide (SMS 201-995). *Clinical Endocrinology* **30:** 385–388.

Wynick D, Ratcliffe WA, Heath DA et al (1990) Treatment of a malignant pancreatic endocrine tumour secreting parathyroid hormone related protein. *British Medical Journal* **300:** 1314–1315.

Zeiger MA, Shawker TH & Norton JA (1993) Use of intraoperative ultrasonography to localize islet cell tumors. *World Journal of Surgery* **17:** 448–454.

Zeitels J, Naunheim K, Kaplan EL & Straus F (1982) Carcinoid tumors: a 37-year experience. *Archives of Surgery* **117:** 732–737.

Zogakis TG & Norton JA (1995) Palliative operations for patients with unresectable endocrine neoplasia. *Surgical Clinics of North America* **75:** 525–538.

9

Gastrointestinal endocrine tumours: medical management

RUDOLF ARNOLD
MARGARETA FRANK

In the management of patients with gastrointestinal endocrine tumours surgery is the only approach to achieve definitive cure of the disease. The most convincing results have been reported from patients with benign and small endocrine tumours (Stefanini et al, 1974; Norton, 1995). In the presence of metastatic spread, surgery might be indicated in the case of, or to prevent bowel obstruction in patients with endocrine tumours of the small and large bowel (Stinner et al, 1996), to reduce tumour masses ('debulking') mostly from the liver (Ahlman et al, 1996) or for liver trans-plantation in patients with tumour spread exclusively limited to the liver (Arnold et al, 1989; Markowka et al, 1989; Alsina et al, 1990; Frilling et al, 1994; Nagorney and Que, 1995). At least in patients with malignant insulinoma, palliative surgery has been repeatedly shown to improve hormone-mediated symptoms and quality of life and to prolong life span in those unresponsive to other medical measures (Figure 1). Therefore, the dialogue between endocrinologists or gastroenterologists and surgeons is a prerequisite in the management of patients with benign and malignant gastrointestinal endocrine tumours. This report summarizes current knowledge of the medical control of hormone-mediated symptoms and of growth of malignant endocrine tumours.

MEDICAL CONTROL OF HORMONE-MEDIATED SYMPTOMS

Gastrointestinal endocrine tumours can be classified according to their site of origin as foregut, midgut and hindgut tumours and according to their secretory product released or not released into circulation into functionally active or inactive tumours. Insulinomas, gastrinomas, VIPomas, most glucagonomas and tumours associated with the carcinoid syndrome are functionally active and their hormonal products frequently threaten a patient's life. Clinical symptoms characteristic of functionally active neuro-endocrine gastroenteropancreatic tumours are listed in Table 1. Control of

Baillière's Clinical Gastroenterology—
Vol. 10, No. 4, December 1996
ISBN 0–7020–2186–5
0950–3528/96/040737 + 23 $12.00/00

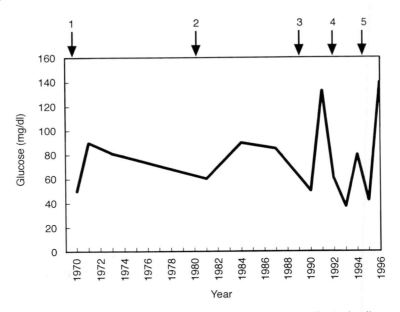

Figure 1. Effect of different therapeutic strategies on the course of a malignant insulinoma first diagnosed in 1970 in a presently 75 year old male patient: 1, partial pancreatectomy; 2, debulking (liver metastases); 3, chemotherapy; 4, chemotherapy and hemihepatectomy; 5, octreotide and chemoembolization of liver metastases.

Table 1. Leading symptoms and medical symptomatic management in patients with gastrointestinal endocrine tumours.

Tumour (syndrome)	Symptoms	Medical symptomatic management
Insulinoma	Neuroglucopenia	Oral, parenteral glucose, diazoxide, somatostatin analogues
Gastrinoma (Zollinger–Ellison syndrome)	Relapsing ulcer disease, diarrhoea, steatorrhoea	Proton-pump inhibitors
VIPoma (Verner–Morrison syndrome, pancreatic cholera)	Watery diarrhoea	Somatostatin analogues
Glucagonoma syndrome	Necrolytic migratory erythema, diabetes mellitus, anaemia	Somatostatin analogues
Somatostatinoma	Diabetes mellitus, steatorrhoea, cholecystolithiasis	Not available
Carcinoid syndrome	Flushing, diarrhoea, abdominal cramping, broncho-obstruction, carcinoid heart disease	Somatostain analogues, serotonin antagonists: cyproheptadine, ketanserine, methysergid, odansetron
Functionally inactive tumours	Local symptoms in the case of large tumours	According to symptoms

mucosal ulcerations can be avoided (Raufman et al, 1983). However, to achieve this extent of acid suppression, basal acid output has to be controlled 1 hour before the next dose of the proton-pump inhibitor. If basal acid output exceeds the criterion of 10 mEq/hour the dose should be doubled with one dose in the morning and the other dose in the evening. This procedure has to be repeated until adequate gastric acid suppression is obtained. In clinical practice, one starts with a morning dose of 40 mg omeprazole or 60 mg lansoprazole or 80 mg pantoprazole. Basal acid output has to be checked 48 hours later and the proton-pump inhibitor dose adjusted accordingly. To avoid over- and underdosing, basal acid output should initially be controlled after 3 months and later at 12 month intervals, since it has been shown that in long-term management the maintenance dose of the proton-pump inhibitor may be too high (Metz et al, 1992) and could be reduced to 20 mg omeprazole daily or twice daily. However, this is not true for patients with concomitant severe reflux disease requiring reduction of gastric acid output to less than 1 mEq/hour to avoid complications of reflux disease such as strictures with the need for subsequent dilatation (Miller et al, 1990).

Somatostatin and its long-acting analogues inhibit gastric acid secretion by a direct effect on the parietal cells and by lowering the release of gastrin from the tumour. They have been, therefore, suggested as an alternative treatment option in the control of gastric acid secretion in gastrinoma patients (Ellison et al, 1986; Ruszniewski et al, 1988; Vinik et al, 1988) (Table 3). Because octreotide and lanreotide must be administered subcutaneously and since octreotide does not in every patient lower acid secretion sufficiently (Koop et al, 1990) this treatment option is superfluous if only control of gastric acid hypersecretion is intended. The same holds true for other antisecretory agents as anti-cholinergics, prostaglandin analogues and surgical vagotomy used prior to the availability of proton-pump inhibitors.

Table 3. Management of gastric acid hypersecretion in gastrinoma patients.

Oral route*		
Omeprazole	20–40 mg once daily ⟶	t.i.d.
Lansoprazole	30–60 mg once daily ⟶	t.i.d.
Pantoprazole†	40–80 mg once daily ⟶	t.i.d.
Parenteral route*		
Omeprazole: 60–100 mg every 12 hours		

* Reduction of basal acid output <10 mEq/hour intended; in patients with concomitant reflux disease <1 mEq/hour.
† At present no prospective studies available on efficacy.

Carcinoid syndrome

The clinical features and treatment options in patients with carcinoid syndrome are summarized in Tables 4 and 5. Although flushing and diarrhoea have been repeatedly reported as the leading symptoms of the disease, they rarely affect patients' well-being and do, therefore, not necessarily require treatment. Performance and general condition can be unrestricted for years despite diffuse liver metastases. First-experienced symptoms of patients with carcinoid syndrome occasionally are signs of right heart failure with dyspnoea and cardiac oedema reflecting the frequently underestimated incidence of cardiac heart disease in 50–70% of patients with the classic carcinoid syndrome (Thorson, 1958; Roberts and Sjoerdsma, 1964; Roberts et al, 1973; Lundin et al 1988, 1990). This is important to recognize because life expectation in these patients is mostly limited by right side heart failure rather than by metastatic disease. Another frequently misinterpreted aspect in patients with carcinoid syndrome concerns diarrhoea. Despite being one of the index symptoms diarrhoea regularly deteriorates after surgical removal of the primary tumour in the terminal ileum by wide segmental resection, by removal of the ileocoecal valve and by ileocolic anastomosis. This could result in bile acid loss and/or increased bacterial contamination of the small intestine with subsequent deconjugation of bile acids. The therapeutic approach in this condition differs from treatment options for hormone-mediated diarrhoea.

Medical management of symptoms derived from the excessive hormone release by the carcinoid tumour and its metastases as flush, diarrhoea, bronchoconstriction and carcinoid crisis has been markedly facilitated by

Table 4. Therapeutic options for patients with cardinoid syndrome.

Symptoms	Proposed mediators	Treatment
Flushing	Tachykinins (neuropeptide K, neuropeptide A, substance P)	Somatostatin analogues Others: α-interferon, avoid alcohol, α-adrenergic blockers, phenothiazine derivatives, glucocorticoids
	Histamine	$H_1 + H_2$ histamine antagonists
	Vasoactive kinine peptides	Somatostatin analogues
Diarrhoea	Serotonin Prostaglandin E, F	Somatostatin analogues Others: parachlorphenylalanine, serotonin antagonists (cyproheptadine, methysergide, odansetron), loperamide, α-interferon
Abdominal cramps	Small bowel obstruction Vascular occlusion mediated by serotonin	Decompression Surgery
Bronchoconstriction	Serotonin Substance P Bradykinins	Somatostatin analogues
Carcinoid heart disease (fibrosis)	Serotonin (?)	Somatostatin analogues? α-Interferon?
Pellagra-like skin symptoms	Niacin deficiency	Niacin supplementation

Table 5. Treatment of patients with carcinoid syndrome.

Flush mediated by tachykinis	Octreotide	50 μg b.i.d. – 200 μg t.i.d. s.c.
	Lanreotide	30 mg every 14 days i.m.
	α-Interferon	3 MIU 3 times weekly s.c.
Flush mediated by histamine	Ranitidine + Astemizol	150 mg t.i.d. + 10 mg t.i.d.
Diarrhoea mediated by	Octreotide	50 μg b.i.d.–200 μg t.i.d. s.c.
hormonal mediators	Lanreotide	30 mg every 14 days i.m.
	Cyproheptadin	4–8 mg t.i.d.
	Methysergide	2 mg b.i.d. – 4 mg t.i.d.
	Odansetron	8 mg b.i.d.
	Loperamide	2 mg t.i.d.
	α-Interferon	3 MI/U three times weekly s.c.
Diarrhoea mediated by		
bile-acid loss	Colestyramine	4 g t.i.d.
bacterial contamination	Doxycyclin	200 mg b.i.d.
Bronchoconstriction	Octreotide	100 μg bid – 200 μg t.i.d. s.c.
	Lanreotide	30 mg every 14 days i.m.
Carcinoid heart disease	Tricuspid and/or pulmonic valve replacement or angioplasty	
	Octreotide ?	
	α-Interferon ?	
Pellagra-like skin symptoms	Nicotinamide	200 mg t.i.d.

the availability of long-acting somatostatin analogues such as octreotide and lanreotide (Tables 4 and 5). Both analogues improve or even normalize diarrhoea and flushing (Kvols et al, 1986; Vinik and Moattari, 1989; Buchanan, 1993; Scherübl et al, 1994; Arnold et al, 1996; Ruszniewski et al, 1996). According to recent studies flushing normalized in 44% or improved in more than 50% of patients during octreotide treatment (Arnold et al, 1996) and resolved completely in 53% of patients during lanreotide treatment (Ruszniewski et al, 1996), during both short- and long-term treatment for 3–12 months. Corresponding figures have been reported for improvement of diarrhoea by octreotide (Arnold et al, 1996), whereas the effect of lanreotide on diarrhoea was less pronounced (Ruszniewski et al, 1996).

Octreotide and lanreotide are well tolerated (Table 6) and discontinuation of treatment is rarely the consequence of side-effects. The most relevant side-effect is the development of gallstones, which is believed to derive from inhibition of gall-bladder emptying due to inhibition of cholecysto-kinine release (Dowling et al, 1992). The precise incidence of newly developed gallstones during long-term treatment with somatostatin analogues is controversial, being reported as up to 60% in the literature. Water intoxication has been described in anecdotal reports (Halma et al, 1987).

Some patients report on worsening of diarrhoea after onset of treatment with long-lasting somatostatin analogues. According to our experiences most of these patients had previously undergone segmental resection of the terminal ileum, removal of the ileocoecal valve and ileocoelic

Table 6. Reported side-effects during treatment with long-acting somatostatin analogues.

Pain at injection site
Flatulence
Diarrhoea
Steatorrhoea
Hyperglycaemia
Gallstones
Alopecia
Water intoxication

---

anastomoses. Diarrhoea in these circumstances frequently improves after administration of anion-binding resins as cholestyramine treatment and dietary substitution of long-chain by medium-chain fatty acids. Bacterial contamination has to be excluded if diarrhoea and/or steatorrhoea persists. Whether or not pancreatic enzyme substitution effects steatorrhoea, also observed in the absence of previous bowel resection (Lembcke et al, 1987), is unsettled.

Only in patients with flushing and diarrhoea refractory to somatostatin analogues should the alternative treatment options (Sjoerdsma et al, 1970; Moertel et al, 1991a) indicated in Tables 4 and 5 be considered. $H_1 + H_2$ histamine receptor antagonists prevent histamine-mediated flushing arising from the very rare gastric carcinoid associated with carcinoid syndrome. Whether specific serotonin antagonists against the five known HT receptors are superior to non-selective antagonists in the treatment of somatostatin-refracting diarrhoea has not been investigated properly (Peart and Robertson, 1961; Gustafsen et al, 1986; Anderson et al 1987; Buhl et al, 1992; von der Ohe et al, 1994).

As well as improving flushing and diarrhoea, the administration of long-acting somatostatin analogues is mandatory to prevent carcinoid crisis including life-threatening bronchial obstruction occurring during laparotomy or during and after embolization of liver metastases. Whether or not carcinoid heart disease can be affected by long-acting somatostatin analogues and/or α-interferon is also unclear.

Pellagra-like lesions often associated with oedema are the consequence of nicotinamide deficiency, which is observed in the case of large tumours. The tumours convert most of the dietary tryptophan to 5-hydroxyindole acetic acid. Nicotinamide therapy has been reported to improve this metabolic imbalance.

α-Interferon also improves flushing and diarrhoea (Di Bartolomeo et al, 1993; Eriksson and Öberg, 1995). Since α-interferons are associated with considerable adverse reactions (Table 7), they should only be recommended if antiproliferative treatment is intended (see below)

Verner–Morrison syndrome

Watery, high-volume diarrhoea (up to 3–10 l of stool per day) with loss of electrolytes and dehydration is the leading symptom in patients with

Table 7. Side-effects during treatment with α-interferons.

Early side-effects	Flu-like symptoms	Nausea
	Diarrhoea	Headaches
	Anorexia	Abdominal cramps
Late side-effects	Decreased libido and/or impotence	
	Chronic fatigue	
	Infections	
	Diarrhoea	
	Elevated liver enzymes	
	Weight loss	
	Hair loss	
	Pancytopenia	
	Pruritic dermatitis	
	Hypertriglyceridaemia with acute pancreatitis	
	Inability to concentrate and short-term memory loss	
	Autoimmune reactions (thyrotoxicosis, vasculitis)	
	Mental depression	

Adapted from Pisegna et al (1993) and Eriksson and Öberg (1995).

Verner–Morrison syndrome. Tumours producing vasoactive intestinal polypeptide (VIP) and peptide histidine methionine (PHM-27) originate mostly from the pancreas and rarely from neural or periganglionic tissue. Malignancy rate is high with metastases mostly to the liver. Somatostatin analogues are currently the therapeutic principle of first choice to control diarrhoea effectively in most but not all patients (Long et al, 1981; Ruskoné et al, 1982; Maton et al, 1985; Santangelo et al, 1985; Wood et al, 1985; O'Dorisio et al, 1989). The mechanism by which somatostatin acts is dual with inhibition of hormonal release from the tumour and direct inhibition of water and electrolyte secretion from the intestine (Ruskoné et al, 1982; Santangelo et al, 1985). Recommended doses are 50–100 μg t.i.d. but some patients need larger doses or have been reported to respond initially to octreotide but to become refractory to octreotide up to 1200 μg per day (Koelz et al, 1987, Maton et al, 1989a; O'Dorisio et al, 1989). Desensitization or receptor downregulation are possible mechanisms behind this rebound phenomenon. In these patients, glucocorticoids (Long et al, 1981; Meckhijan and O'Dorisio 1987), indomethacin (Jaffe et al, 1977), lithium (Pandol et al, 1980), surgical tumour debulking, hepatic artery embolization or chemotherapy should be considered as adjuncts or alternatively. Although current experiences are based on octreotide, lanreotide is expected to be effective as well in Verner–Morrison syndrome in a dosage of 30 mg every other week.

Glucagonoma syndrome

Tumour debulking including resection of the primary and of its metastases should be performed, wherever possible, to reduce plasma glucagone and, by this, to improve the necrolytic migratory erythema, protein hyper-catabolism and hypoacidonaemia. As an adjunct or if tumour debulking is impossible, long-acting somatostatin analogues have been shown to be effective (Kessinger et al, 1977; Long et al, 1979; Anderson and Bloom, 1986; Boden et al, 1986; Ch'ng et al, 1986; Kvols et al, 1987; Rosenbaum et al, 1989). According to these studies complete disappearance of cutaneous lesions is rare but improvement can be achieved in 50–90% of patients. The control of cutaneous symptoms is parallelled by restoration of the nutritional status, regaining weight and resolution of diarrhoea. In most studies, 100–400 µg/day of octreotide at two or three divided doses have been used. Some patients needed higher doses or became refractory after initial response. In these patients, chemotherapy or other strategies to reduce tumour volume have to be considered.

MEDICAL CONTROL OF TUMOUR GROWTH

Therapeutic strategies for the control of tumour growth in patients with metastatic gastrointestinal tumours must keep in mind the spontaneous tumour growth, which varies from one patient to another. Some tumours remain unchanged in size for months or even years without therapy, others grow slowly, independently of any antiproliferative measures, and still others exhibit exploding growth (Creutzfeldt, 1985; Arnold et al, 1993). Taking into account the severe side-effects of currently available chemotherapeutic protocols with unproven efficacy in patients with slowly growing tumours, chemotherapy is not indicated in the latter group of patients. Aggressive antiproliferative strategies are only desired in fast-growing tumours and in patients where the severity of the associated endocrine syndrome (carcinoid syndrome; glucagonoma syndrome) is unresponsive to less harmful therapeutic measures (Arnold et al, 1993; Moertel, 1993). In general, therapeutic strategies in the control of tumour growth include several options: surgical measures such as tumour debulking (Rothmund et al, 1991), embolization of the hepatic artery (Allison et al, 1985; Carrasco et al, 1986), treatment with long-acting somatostatin analogues, interferon α (IFNα), combination of somatostatin analogues and IFNα, systemic chemotherapy and, in selective patients, liver transplantation (Markowka et al, 1989).

Because of the low incidence of gastrointestinal endocrine tumours, only few controlled studies are available in which the effect of specific therapeutic measures has been investigated prospectively. Even in these studies tumours of different origins (foregut, midgut, hindgut; pancreatic, intestinal) have been pooled. Currently available antiproliferative strategies based on larger, prospective studies will be analysed in the following sections.

Long-acting somatostatin analogues

Evidence for additional antiproliferative properties arises from in vitro data using tumour cell lines, from animal models with solid tumours (Schally, 1988; Liebow et al, 1989; Hofland et al, 1992; Buscail et al,

1994) and from case reports describing even tumour regression in patients with metastatic gastrointestinal endocrine tumours (Kraenzlin et al, 1983; Clements and Elias, 1985; Shepherd and Senator, 1986; Wiedenmann et al, 1988; Creutzfeldt et al, 1991). Two prospective studies are available which addressed the antiproliferative effect of octreotide on tumour growth. They confirmed the beneficial effect on hormone-mediated symptoms and, in addition, could show that octreotide indeed inhibits tumour growth in 50% (Saltz et al, 1993) or 36% (Arnold et al, 1996) of patients. The most favourable response was stabilization of tumour growth after CT-documented tumour progression prior to treatment. Tumour regression has not been observed in both prospective studies. Octreotide doses ranged between 150 and 250 µg octreotide t.i.d. with no further beneficial effect in those patients treated with up to 500 µg octreotide t.i.d. (Arnold et al, 1996). Although median duration of stable disease was 18 months, the antiproliferative effect of octreotide was, at least in some patients, long lasting. Patients with a good Karnofsky performance score and those with tumours originating from the small intestine or with carcinoid syndrome responded better than patients with pancreatic tumours. In a subgroup of patients with stable disease prior to octreotide treatment stable disease continued in 54% of patients over more than 12 months. It could not be elucidated whether this effect mirrors the spontaneous course of the disease or a possibly beneficial antiproliferative effect of octreotide (Arnold et al, 1996). Lanreotide has not been investigated with respect to growth inhibition of gastrointestinal endocrine tumours so far. Recently, it has been shown that inhibition of cell proliferation by somatostatin analogues is mediated by the receptor subtypes sst_2 and sst_5 (Buscail et al, 1994). However, this has to be further investigated in endocrine tumours. Whether or not octreotide prolongs life expectancy cannot be concluded from available studies. Nevertheless, octreotide seems to be an effective therapeutic option in patients with slowly growing tumours and is accompanied by fewer side-effects than the strategies discussed below.

Interferons

The mechanisms by which interferons affect tumour growth have not been elucidated. IFNα blocked the cell cycle of cells derived from a human carcinoid tumour during the G_0–G_1 phase with prolongation of the S phase (Öberg, 1994). Some data suggest that IFNα induces apoptosis and that tumour cells are replaced by fibrotic tissue. This could explain the increased intratumoral fibrosis observed in metastases of endocrine tumours without a significant change in tumour size (Anderson et al, 1990). IFNα further induces increased expression of class I antigenes on the tumour cell surface which renders cells as targets for cytotoxic T lymphocytes.

Several studies of the antiproliferative effect of IFNα in patients with metastatic pancreatic and intestinal endocrine tumours have been reported (Öberg et al, 1986; Smith et al, 1987; Hanssen et al, 1989; Moertel et al, 1989; Di Bartolomeo et al, 1993; Pisegna et al, 1993; Öberg et al, 1994;

Eriksson and Öberg, 1995). According to these experiences 40–50% of patients respond biochemically with a greater than 50% reduction of the index hormone and an concomitant improvement of flushing and diarrhoea in patients with carcinoid syndrome. Stabilization of tumour growth was observed in 20–40%, and a reduction in tumour size in 12–20% of patients (Moertel et al, 1986; Eriksson and Öberg, 1995). In the Moertel study including patients with carcinoid syndrome, the favourable trend was transient in nature, with hormonal responses and objective regression persisting for a mean of only 7 weeks. In accordance with this study are observations in patients with metastatic gastrinoma (Pisegna et al, 1993). In contrast, Swedish investigators reported a median duration of response lasting between 16 and 20 months (Eriksson and Öberg, 1995). If interferon is considered as first-line antiproliferative therapy, its questionable therapeutic gain shown by the majority of available reports must be out-weighed by the frequency and severity of toxic reactions (Table 7). Interesting are the few reports on the combination of octreotide with IFNα (Joenssuu, et al, 1992; Nold et al, 1994). Both studies indicate that the combination might be superior to monotherapy with either substances. Prospective studies are currently under way to investigate the effect of long-acting somatostatin analogues and IFNα as monotherapy versus the combination of both principles.

Chemotherapy

Reports on the effect of chemotherapy on tumour growth and survival in patients with advanced metastatic gastrointestinal endocrine tumours are numerous and have been extensively reviewed recently (Kvols and Buck, 1987; Arnold and Frank, 1995).

Chemotherapy reached a new therapeutic dimension after the purification of streptozotocin derived from a fermentation of broth of *Streptomyces achromogenes*. The name streptozotocin takes into account its *Streptomyces* origin and its azo, or nitrogen-containing, chemical structure. During pre-clinical studies it became apparent that streptozotocin, which was purified during a search for new antimicrobial agents, produced hyperglycaemia in rats and dogs within a few hours (Rakieten et al, 1963). Streptozotocin was first used in the treatment of patients with a multiple-hormone-producing metastatic islet cell tumour resulting in an objective decrease of both measurable tumour and hormone production (Murray-Lyon et al, 1968). Since these reports, one of the ascertained indications for streptozotocin in combination with 5-fluorouracil (Table 8) has been symptomatic and antiproliferative treatment of patients with metastatic insulinoma (Creutzfeldt, 1995). Subsequent reports on the effect of strepto-zotocin on metastatic gastrointestinal tumours were inconclusive and often hampered by studies (a) involving mostly a handful of cases, (b) revealing varied criteria employed for assessing response, (c) involving tumours of various origin and (d) neglecting the varying malignant potentials of metastatic endocrine tumours which could differ between well-differen-tiated and undifferentiated tumours (Moertel et al, 1980; Johnson et al,

Table 8. Systemic chemotherapy: well-differentiated metastatic islet-cell tumours.

(1) Streptozocin	500 mg/m^2 as intravenous injection for 5 consecutive days
Doxorublcin	50 mg/m^2 as intravenous injection on days 1 and 22; repeated every 6 weeks
(2) Streptozocin	500 mg/m^2 as intravenous injection for 5 consecutive days
5-Fluorouracil	400 mg/m^2 as intravenous injection for 5 consecutive days; repeated every 6 weeks

Maximal dose of doxorubicin: 500 mg/m^2. Reduced dosages of every drug in case of severe nausea, vomiting, stomatitis, diarrhoea, leucopenia, thrombocytopenia. Reduced dosages of streptozocin in case of elevated creatinine or proteinaemia and discontinuation if abnormalities persist. Adopted from Moertel et al (1992).

1983; Shridhar et al, 1985; Kvols and Buck, 1987; Moertel et al, 1991b). More recent studies acknowledged at least some of these prerequisites. The Eastern Cooperatve Oncology Group investigated prospectively three regimens in patients with histologically proved, unresectable islet carcinomas and found that the combination of streptozotocin plus doxorubicin was superior to streptozotocin plus 5-fluorouracil and to chlorozotocin (Moertel et al, 1992). Tumour regression was observed in 69% of the patients on streptozotocin plus doxorubicin, in 45% of patients on streptozotocin plus 5-fluorouracil, and in 30% of patients treated with chlorozotocin alone. Median durations of regression were 18 months for the doxorubicin versus 14 months for the fluorouracil combination and 17 months for chlorozotocin monotherapy. Survival time was also beneficially influenced. As expected, toxic reactions including long-lasting nausea, vomiting, haematological toxicity, leukopenia, cardiomyopathy and renal insufficiency were observed as major side-effects. These encouraging findings could not be confirmed in a very homogenous study group including 10 patients with metastatic gastrinoma (von Schrenck et al, 1988). Therefore, the significance of the data reported by the Eastern Cooperative Oncology Group remains unsettled.

Various single agents such as doxorubicin, 5-fluorouracil, DTIC, mitomycin and others as well as drug combinations including streptozotocin have been tested in patients with endocrine tumours arising from the intestine, i.e. those with malignant carcinoid syndrome (Engström et al, 1984; Moertel, 1993). The authors concluded that no chemotherapy regimen currently provides an appropriate standard therapy for this disease and can, therefore, only be offered on an experimental basis.

In contrast to patients with well-differentiated carcinoids, those with anaplastic neuroendocrine carcinoma might benefit from chemotherapy. Anaplastic neuroendocrine carcinoma is characterized by a histologically less well developed neuroendocrine pattern, greater cytological atypia than carcinoid tumours, greater mitotic activity, and small foci of necrosis (Moertel et al, 1991b). These histological characteristics are associated with a more rapid advance of malignant disease and, less frequently, clinically recognizable excess hormone production. The tumours have been observed to originate from the small and large bowel, pancreas and stomach. In a study performed in 18 patients with anaplastic neuroendocrine tumours and in 13 patients with well-differentiated carcinoid tumours and in 14 patients with malignant islet cell tumours the effect of a regimen of etoposide plus cisplatin (Table 9) was investigated (Moertel et al, 1991b). Among 13 patients with well differentiated carcinoid tumour, none showed an objective tumour response or alleviation of clinical symptoms. Among the 14 patients with metastatic islet cell carcinoma, two (15%) had partial tumour regression lasting for 4.5 to 6.0 months. In contrast, an objective tumour response was observed in 12 of 18 patients (67%) with anaplastic neuroendocrine carcinoma. Three tumours responded completely and eight partially. The median duration of regression was 8 months (range 3–21 months). The interval to progression ranged from 2 to 21 months. Thus, the overall regression rate of patients with anaplastic neuroendocrine carcinoma was similar to that observed for extensive small-cell lung cancer. Drug toxicity included nausea, vomiting, sensory neuropathy, alopecia, leukopenia, thrombocytopenia and renal insufficiency.

Table 9. Systemic chemotherapy: fast-growing, anaplastic neuroendocrine carcinoids.

Etoposide	130 mg/m^2 as 24 hour intravenous infusion for 3 consecutive days
Cisplatin	45 mg/m^2 as 24 hour intravenous infusion on days 2 and 3

Repeated every 4 weeks. Reduction in dose in case of excessive toxicity during the proceeding course.
Add appropriate anti-emetics.
Adapted from Moertel et al (1991).

SUMMARY

With the introduction of longer-acting somatostatin analogues symptomatic relief is easy to achieve in patients with functionally active endocrine tumours and will be further facilitated by still longer-acting formulations. The consequences of gastric acid hypersecretion in patients with Zollinger–Ellison syndrome can be prevented by all proton-pump inhibitors currently on the market.

Despite the various antiproliferative strategies that have been offered to patients with metastatic disease, available data are controversial and, more importantly, are supported by few prospective and controlled studies. Most experts agree that surgery with curative extirpation of the primary in the absence of metastases and tumour debulking in metastatic disease should be intended wherever possible. Controversy concerns residual disease. According to our view, any further antiproliferative strategy should consider the growth characteristics and biology of a given tumour (Figure 4). In the case of rapid progression, chemotherapy should be offered if tumours originate from the pancreas or reveal an undifferentiated histology. In contrast, chemotherapy should not be offered to patients with well-differentiated non-functional or functional tumours (carcinoid syndrome) arising from the intestine. The same applies for patients with tumours with no or only slow growth within an given observation period of 3–12 months. These patients should be treated only symptomatically.

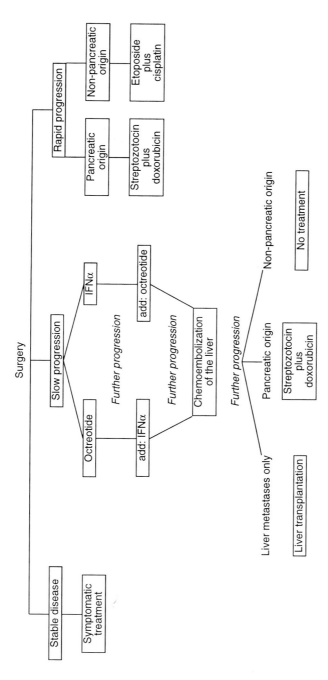

Figure 4. Antiproliferative treatment options in metastatic gastrointestinal tumours.

Patients with tumours of slow progression might favourably respond to long-acting somatostatin analogues. We start with octreotide and offer patients not responding to octreotide monotherapy additional IFNα. If further tumour progression takes place, hepatic artery embolization is the next step (Figure 5) followed by chemotherapy, the latter in patients with tumours of pancreatic origin only. This strategy recognizes the severity of side-effects of the different therapeutic modalities and starts with octreotide because of its very few side-effects. Other groups start with chemo-embolization followed by octreotide, α-interferon or its combinations (Ahlman et al, 1996). Ongoing studies will, it is hoped, answer the question of the ideal sequence of therapeutic strategies. Every available patient with metastasised gastrointestinal endocrine tumours should be included in one of the ongoing European multicentre trials.

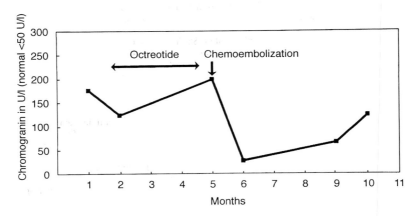

Figure 5. Chromogranin A plasma levels in a patient with metastatic non-functioning neuroendocrine tumour not responding to octreotide but to chemoembolization of hepatic metastases.

REFERENCES

Ahlman H, Westberg G, Wängberg B (1996) Treatment of liver metastases of carcinoid tumors. *World Journal of Surgery* **20:** 196–202.

Allison DJ, Jordan H & Hennessy O (1985) Therapeutic embolization of the hepatic artery: a review of 75 procedures. *Lancet* **i:** 595–599.

Alsina AE, Bartus S, Hull D et al (1990) Liver transplantation for metastatic neuroendocrine tumors. *Journal of Clinical Gastroenterology* **12:** 535–537.

Anderson JV & Bloom SR (1986) Neuroendocrine tumours of the gut: long-term therapy with the somatostatin analogue SMS 201-995. *Scandinavian Journal of Gastroenterology* **21 (supplement 119):** 115–128.

Anderson JV, Coups MO, Morris JA et al (1987) Remission of symptoms in carcinoid syndrome with a new 5-hydroxytryptamine M receptor antagonist. *British Medical Journal* **294:** 1129.

Anderson T, Wilander E, Eriksson B et al (1990) Effects of interferon on tumor tissue content in liver metastases of carcinoid tumors. *Cancer Research* **50:** 3413–3415.

Arnold R (1990) Therapeutic strategies in the management of endocrine GEP tumours. *European Journal of Clinical Investigation* **20 (supplement 1):** 82–90.

Arnold R & Frank M (1995) Systemic chemotherapy for endocrine tumors of the pancreas: recent advances. In Mignon M & Jensen RT (eds) *Endocrine Tumors of the Pancreas, Frontiers of Gastrointestinal Research*, vol. 23, pp 431–438. Basel: Karger.

Arnold JC, O'Grady JG, Bird GL et al (1989) Liver transplantation for primary and secondary hepatic apudomas. *British Journal of Surgery* **76:** 248–249.

Arnold R, Neuhaus C, Benning R et al (1993) Somatostatin analog Sandostatin and inhibition of tumor growth in patients with metastatic endocrine gastroenteropancreatic tumors. *World Journal of Surgery* **17:** 511–519

Arnold R, Trautmann ME, Creutzfeldt W et al (1996) Somatostatin analogue octreotide and inhibition of tumour growth in metastatic endocrine gastroenteropancreatic tumors. *Gut* **38:** 430–438.

Boden G, Ryan IG, El Senschmid BL et al (1986) Treatment of inoperable glucagonoma with the long-acting somatostatin analogue SMS 201-995. *New England Journal of Medicine* **314:** 1686–1689.

Buchanan KD (1993) Effects of sandostatin on neuroendocrine tumors of the gastrointestinal system. *Recent Results in Cancer Research* **129:** 45–55.

Buhl C, Fibbe C & Frenzel H (1992) Ondansetron in carcinoid syndrome. *Deutsche Medizinische Wochenschrift* **117:** 1821.

Buscail L, Delesque N, Esteve JP et al (1994) Stimulation of tyrosine phosphatase and inhibition of cell proliferation by somatostatin analogues: mediation by human somatostatin receptor subtypes SSTR1 and SSTR2. *Proceedings of the National Academy of Sciences of the USA* **91:** 2315–2319.

Carrasco CH, Charnsangavej Ch, Ajani J et al (1986) The carcinoid syndrome: palliation by hepatic artery embolization. *American Journal of Radiology* **147:** 149–154.

Ch'ng JL, Anderson JV, Williams SJ et al (1986) Remission of symptoms during long term treatment of metastatic pancreatic endocrine tumours with long-acting somatostatin analogue. *British Medical Journal* **292:** 981–982.

Clements D & Elias E (1985) Regression of metastatic VIPoma with somatostatin analogue SMS 201-995. *Lancet* **i:** 874–875.

Collen MJ, Howard JM, McArthur KE et al (1984) Comparison of ranitidine and cimetidine in the treatment of gastric hypersecretion. *Annals of Internal Medicine* **100:** 52–58.

Comi RJ, Gorden P & Doppmann JL (1993) In Go VLW et al (eds) *The Pancreas: Biology and Disease*, 2nd edn, pp 979–997. New York: Raven Press.

Creutzfeldt W (1985) Endocrine tumours of the pancreas. In Arquilla E & Volks BW (eds) *The Diabetic Pancreas*, pp 543–563. New York: Plenum

Creutzfeldt W (1995) Insulinomas: clinical presentation, diagnosis and advances in management. In Mignon M & Jensen RT (eds) *Endocrine Tumors of the Pancreas, Frontiers of Gastrointestinal Research*, vol. 23, pp 148–165. Basel: Karger.

Creutzfeldt W, Arnold R, Creutzfeldt C et al (1974) Biochemical and morphological investigation in 30 human insulinomas. *Diabetologia* **9:** 217–231.

Creutzfeldt W, Bartsch HH, Jacubaschke U et al (1991) Treatment of gastrointestinal endocrine tumors with interferon-alpha and octreotide. *Acta Oncologica* **30:** 529–535.

Di Bartolomeo M, Bajetta E, Zilembo N et al (1993) Treatment of carcinoid syndrome with recombinant interferon alpha-2a. *Acta Oncologica* **32:** 235–238.

Dowling RH, Hussaini SH, Murphy GM et al (1992) Gallstones during octreotide therapy. *Metabolism* **41 (supplement 2):** 22–33.

Ellison EC, O'Dorisio TH & Woltering EA (1986) Suppression of gastrin and gastric acid secretion in the Zollinger–Ellison syndrome by long-acting somatostatin. *Scandinavian Journal of Gastroenterology* **21:** 206–211.

Engström PF, Lavin PT, Moertel CG et al (1984) Streptozotocin plus fluorouracil versus doxorubicin therapy for metastatic carcinoid tumors. *Journal of Clinical Oncology* **3:** 1255–1259.

Eriksson B & Öberg K (1995) Interferon therapy of malignant endocrine pancretic tumors. In Mignon M & Jensen RT (eds) *Endocrine Tumors of the Pancreas, Frontiers of Gastrointestinal Research*, vol. 23, pp 451–460. Basel: Karger.

Frerichs H & Track NS (1974) Pharmacotherapy of hormone-secreting tumors. *Clinics in Gastroenterology* **3:** 721–732.

Frilling A, Rogiers K, Knöfel WT & Broelsch CE (1994) Liver transplantation for metastic carcinoid tumours. *Digestion* **55 (supplement 3):** 104–106.

Frucht H, Maton PN & Jensen RT (1991) The use of omeprazole in patients with Zollinger–Ellison syndrome. *Digestive Diseases Sciences* **36:** 394–404.

Gustafsen J, Rendorf A, Raskor H & Boesby S (1986) Ketanserin versus placebo in carcinoid syndrome. *Scandinavian Journal of Gastroenterology* **21**: 816–818.

Halma C, Jansen JB, Janssens R et al (1987) Life-threatening water intoxication during somatostatin therapy. *Annals of Internal Medicine* **107**: 518–520.

Hanssen LE, Schrumpf E, Kolbenstredt AN et al (1989) Recombinant alpha-2 interferon with or without hepatic artery embolization in the treatment of midgut carcinoid tumours—a preliminary report. *Acta Oncologica* **28**: 439–443.

Hofland LJ, van Koetsveld PM, Wouters N et al (1992) Dissociation of antiproliferative and antihormonal effects of the somatostatin analog octreotide on 7315b pituitary tumor cells. *Endocrinology* **131**: 571–577.

Jaffe BM, Kopen DF, De Schryver-Kecskemeti K et al (1977) Indomethacin-responsive pancreatic cholera. *New England Journal of Medicine* **297**: 817–821.

Joensuu H, Kätka K & Kujari H (1992) Dramatic response of a metastatic carcinoid tumour to a combination of interferon and octreotide. *Acta Endocrinologica (Copenhagen)* **126**: 184–185.

John M, Meyerhof W, Richter D et al (1996) Positive somatostatin receptor scintigraphy correlates with the presence of somatostatin receptor subtypes 2 and 5. *Gut* **38**: 33–39.

Johnson LA, Lavin P, Moertel CG et al (1983) Carcinoids: the association of histologic growth pattern and survival. *Cancer* **51**: 882–889.

Kessinger A, Lemon HM & Foley JF (1977) The glucagonoma syndrome and its management. *Journal of Surgical Oncology* **9**: 419–424.

Koelz A, Kraenzlin M, Gyr K et al (1987) Escape of the response to a long-acting somatostatin analogue (SMS 201-995) in patients with VIPoma. *Gastroenterology* **92**: 527–531.

Koop H, Klein M & Arnold R (1990) Acid inhibitory effects of somatostatin analog in malignant gastrinoma. *Journal of Clinical Gastroenterology* **12**: 120–121.

Kraenzlin ME, Ch'ng JC, Wood SM & Bloom SR (1983) Can inhibition of hormone secretion be associated with endocrine tumour shrinkage. *Lancet* **ii**: 1501–1504.

Kubota A, Yamada Y, Kagimoto S et al (1994) Identification of somatostatin receptor subtypes and an implication for the efficacy of somatostatin analogue SMS 201-995 in treatment of human endocrine tumors. *Journal of Clinical Investigation* **93**: 1321–1325.

Kvols LK & Buck M (1987) Chemotherapy of endocrine malignancies: a review. *Seminars in Oncology* **14**: 343–383.

Kvols LK, Moertel CG, O'Connel MJ et al (1986) Treatment of the malignant carcinoid syndrome: evaluation of a long-acting somatostatin analogue. *New England Journal of Medicine* **315**: 663–666.

Kvols LK, Buck M, Moertel CG et al (1987) Treatment of metastatic islet cell carcinoma with a somatostatin analogue (SMS 201-995). *Annals of Internal Medicine* **107**: 162–168.

Lamberts SWS, Uitterlinden P, Verschoor L et al (1985) Long-term treatment of acromegaly with the somatostatin analogue SMS 202-995. *New England Journal of Medicine* **313**: 1576–1579.

Lembcke B, Creutzfeldt W, Schleser S et al (1987) Effect of somatostatin analogue sandostatin (SMS 201-996) on gastrointestinal, pancreatic and biliary function and hormone release in normal men. *Digestion* **36**: 108–124.

Liebow C, Reilly C, Serrano M & Schally AV (1989) Somatostatin analogues inhibit growth of pancreatic cancer by stimulating tyrosine phosphatase. *Proceedings of the National Academy of Sciences of the USA* **86**: 2003–2007.

Long RG, Adrian TE, Brown MR et al (1979) Suppression of a pancreatic endocrine tumour secretion by long-acting somatostatin analogue. *Lancet* **ii**: 764–767.

Long RG, Bryant MG, Michell SJ et al (1981) Clinicopathological study of pancreatic and ganglio-neuroblastoma tumours secreting vasoactive intestinal polypeptide (Vipomas). *British Medical Journal* **282**: 1767–1771.

Lundin L, Norheim L, Lundelius J et al (1988) Carcinoid heart disease: relationship of circulating vasoactive substances to ultrasound-detectable cardiac abnormalities. *Circulation* **77**: 264–269.

Lundin L, Hansson HE, Lundelius J & Öberg K (1990) Surgical treatment of carcinoid heart disease. *Journal of Thoracic and Cardiovascular Surgery* **100**: 558–561.

Markowka L, Tzakis AG, Mazzaferro V et al (1989) Transplantation of the liver for metastatic endocrine tumors of the intestine and pancreas. *Surgical Gynecology and Obstetrics* **168**: 107–111.

Maton PN, O'Dorisio TM, Howe BA et al (1985) Effect of long-acting somatostatin analogue (SMS 201-995) in a patient with pancreatic cholera. *New England Journal of Medicine* **312**: 17–21.

Maton PN, Gardner JD & Jensen RT (1989a) Use of long-acting somatostatin analogue SMS 201-995 in patients with pancreatic islet cell tumors. *Digestive Disease Sciences* **34 (supplement):** 285–291.

Maton PN, Vinayek R, Frucht H et al (1989b) Long-term efficacy and safety of omeprazole in patients with Zollinger–Ellison syndrome: a prospective study. *Gastroenterology* **97:** 827–836.

McArthur KE, Collen MJ, Maton PN et al (1985) Omeprazole: effective convenient therapy for Zollinger–Ellison syndrome. *Gastroenterology* **88:** 939–944.

McCarthy DM (1978) Report on the United States experience with cimetidine in Zollinger–Ellison syndrome and other hypersecretory states. *Gastroenterology* **74:** 453–458.

Meckhijan HS & O'Dorisio TM (1987) Vipoma syndrome. *Seminars in Oncology* **14:** 282–291.

Metz DC & Jensen RT (1995) Advances in gastric antisecretory therapy in Zollinger–Ellison-syndrome. In Mignon M & Jensen RT (eds) *Endocrine Tumours of the Pancreas, Frontiers of Gastrointestinal Research*, vol. 23, pp 240–257. Basel: Karger.

Metz DC, Pisegna JR, Fishbeyn VA et al (1992) Current maintenance doses of omeprazole in Zollinger–Ellison syndrome are too high. *Gastroenterology* **103:** 1498–1508.

Metz DC, Pisegna JR, Ringham GL et al (1993) Prospective study of the efficacy and safety of lansoprazole in Zollinger–Ellison syndrome. *Digestive Disease Sciences* **38:** 245–256.

Miller CS, Vinayek R, Frucht H et al (1990) Reflux esophagitis in patients with Zollinger–Ellison syndrome. *Gastroenterology* **98:** 341–346.

Moertel CG (1993) Gastrointetinal carcinoid tumors and the malignant carcinoid syndrome. In Sleisenger MH & Fordtran JS (eds) *Gastrointestinal Disease*, 5th edn, pp 1363–1378. Philadelphia, PA: Saunders.

Moertel CG, Hanley JA & Johnson LA (1980) Streptozotocin alone compared with streptozotocin plus fluorouracil in the treatment of advanced islet-cell carcinoma. *New England Journal of Medicine* **303:** 1189–1194.

Moertel CG, Rubin J & O'Connell MJ (1986) Phase II study of cisplatin therapy in patients with metastatic carcinoid tumor and the malignant carcinoid syndrome. *Cancer Treatment Reports* **70:** 1459–1460.

Moertel CG, Rubin J & Kvols LK (1989) Therapy of metastatic carcinoid tumor and the malignant carcinoid syndrome with recombinant leukocyte A interferon. *Journal of Clinical Oncology* **7:** 865–868.

Moertel CG, Kvols LK & Rubin J (1991a) A study of cyproheptadine in the treatment of metastatic carcinoid tumor and the malignant carcinoid syndrome. *Cancer* **67:** 33–36.

Moertel CG, Kvols LK, O'Connell MJ & Rubin J (1991b) Treatment of neuroendocrine carcinomas with combined etoposide and cisplatin. Evidence of major therapeutic activity in the anaplastic variants of these neoplasms. *Cancer* **68:** 227–232.

Moertel CG, Lefkopoulo M, Lipsitz S et al (1992) Streptozotocin–doxorubicin, streptozotocin–fluorouracil, or chlorozotocin in the treatment of advanced islet-cell carcinoma. *New England Journal of Medicine* **326:** 519–523.

Morange I, De Boisvilliers F, Chanson P et al (1994) Slow release lanreotide treatment in acromegalic patients previously normalized by octreotide. *Journal of Clinicial Endocrinology and Metabolism* **79:** 145–151.

Murray-Lyon IM, Eddleston ALWF, Williams R et al (1968) Treatment of multiple-hormone-producing malignant islet-cell tumour with streptozotocin. *Lancet* **ii:** 895–898.

Nagorney DM & Que FG (1995) Cytoreductive hepatic surgery for metastatic gastrointestinal neuro-endocrine tumors. In Mignon M & Jensen RT (eds) *Endocrine Tumors of the Pancreas, Frontiers of Gastrointestinal Research*, vol. 23, pp 416–430. Basel: Karger.

Nauck M, Stöckmann F & Creutzfeldt W (1990) Evaluation of a euglycaemic clamp procedure as a diagnostic test in insulinoma patients. *European Journal of Clinical Investigation* **20:** 15–28.

Nold R, Frank M, Kajdan U et al (1994) Kombinierte Behandlung metastasierter endokriner Tumoren des Gastrointestinaltrakts mit Octreotid und Interferon-Alpha. *Zeitschrift für Gastroenterologie* **32:** 193–197.

Norton JA (1995) Surgical treatment of islet cell tumours with special emphasis on operative ultra-sound. In Mignon M & Jensen RT (eds) *Endocrine Tumors of the Pancreas, Frontiers of Gastrointestinal Research*, vol. 23, pp 309–332. Basel: Karger.

O'Dorisio TM, Mekhjan H & Gaginella TS (1989) Medical therapy of VIPomas. *Endocrinology Clinics of North America* **18:** 545–556.

Öberg K, Nordheim I, Lind E et al (1986) Treatment of malignant carcinoid tumours with human leucocyte interferon: long-term results. *Cancer Treatment and Research* **70:** 1297–1304.

Öberg K, Eriksson B & Tiensuu Janson E (1994) Interferons alone or in combination with chemotherapy or other biologicals in the treatment of neuroendocrine gut and pancreatic tumors.
Digestion 55 (supplement 3): 64–69.

Pandol SJ, Korman LY, McCarthy DM & Gardner JD (1980) Beneficial effects of oral lithium
carbonate in the treatment of pancreatic cholera syndrome. *New England Journal of Medicine*
302: 1403–1404.

Patel YC & Srikant CB (1994) Subtype selectivity of peptide analogs for all five cloned human
somatostatin receptors (hsstr 1–5). *Endocrinology* 135: 2814–2817.

Peart WS & Robertson JIS (1961) The effect of a serotonin antagonist (UML491) in carcinoid disease.
Lancet 2: 1172–1174.

Pisegna JR, Slimak GG, Doppman JL et al (1993) An evaluation of human recombinant α interferon
in patients with metastatic gastrinoma. *Gastroenterology* 105: 1179–1183.

Plewe G, Beyer J, Krause U et al (1984) Long-acting and selective suppression of growth-hormone
secretion by somatostatin analogue SMS 201-995 in acromegaly. *Lancet* 2: 782–784.

Rakieten N, Rakieten ML & Nadkarni MV (1963) Studies on the diabetogenic action of streptozotocin
(NSC-37919). *Cancer Chemotherapy Reports* 29: 91–98.

Raufman JP, Collins SM, Pandol S et al (1983) Reliability of symptoms in assessing control of gastric
acid secretion in patients with Zollinger–Ellison syndrome. *Gastroenterology* 84: 108–113.

Roberts WC & Sjoerdsma A (1964) The cardiac disease associated with the carcinoid syndrome
(carcinoid heart disease). *American Journal of Medicine* 36: 5–34.

Roberts WC, Dangel JC & Bulkley BGC (1973) Non-rheumatic valvular cardiac disease: a clinicopathologic survey of 27 different conditions causing valvular dysfunction. *Cardiovascular
Clinics* 5: 333–446.

Rosenbaum A, Flourie B, Chagnon S et al (1989) Octreotide (SMS 201-995) in the treatment of
metastatic glucagonoma: report of one case and review of the literature. *Digestion* 42:
116–120.

Rothmund M, Stinner B & Arnold R (1991) Endocrine pancreatic carcinoma. *European Journal of
Surgical Oncology* 17: 191–199.

Ruskoné A, René E, Chayvialle JA et al (1982) Effect of somatostatin on diarrhea and on small
intestinal water and electrolyte transport in a patient with pancreatic cholera. *Digestive Diseases
Sciences* 27: 459–466.

Ruszniewski P, Laucournet H, Elounar-Blanc L et al (1988) Long-acting somatostatin (SMS 201-995)
in the management of Zollinger–Ellison syndrome: evidence for sustained efficacy. *Pancreas* 3:
145–152.

Ruszniewski P, Ducreux M, Chayvialle JA et al (1996) Treatment of the carcinoid syndrome with the
longacting somatostatin analogue lanreotide: a prospective study in 39 patients. *Gut* 39:
279–283.

Saltz L, Trochanowsky G, Buckley M et al (1993) Octreotide as an anti-neoplastic agent in the treatment of functional and non-functional neuroendocrine tumours. *Cancer* 72: 244–248.

Santangelo WC, O'Dorisio TM, Kim JG et al (1985) Pancreatic cholera syndrome: effect of a synthetic somatostatin analog on intestinal water and ion transport. *Annals of Internal Medicine* 103:
363–367.

Schally AV (1988) Oncological application of somatostatin analogues. *Cancer Research* 48:
6977–6985 (Schally AV (1989) *Cancer Research* 49: 1618 (erratum)).

Scherübl H, Wiedenmann B, Riecken EO et al (1994) Treatment of the carcinoid syndrome with a
depot formulation of the somatostatin analogue lanreotide. *European Journal of Cancer* 10:
1591–1592.

Shepherd JJ & Senator GB (1986) Regression of liver metastases in patient with gastrin-secreting
tumour treated with SMS 201-995. *Lancet* ii: 574.

Sjoerdsma A, Lovenberg W & Engelman K (1970) Serotonin now; clinical implications of inhibiting
its synthesis with parachlorphenylalanine. *Annals of Internal Medicine* 73: 607–629.

Shridhar KS, Holland JF, Brown JC et al (1985) Doxorubicin plus cisplatin in the treatment of
apudomas. *Cancer* 55: 2634–2637.

Smith DB, Scarffe JH, Wagstaff J & Johnston RJ (1987) Phase II trial of rDNA alpha 2b interferon in
patients with malignant carcinoid tumour. *Cancer Treatment Reviews* 7: 1265–1266.

Stefanini P, Carboni M & Patrussi N (1974) Surgical treatment and prognosis of insulinoma. *Clinics
in Gastroenterology* 3: 697–712.

Stinner B, Kisker O, Zielke A & Rothmund M (1996) Surgical management for carcinoid tumors of
small bowel, appendix, colon and rectum. *World Journal of Surgery* 20: 183–188.

Thorson AH (1958) Studies on carcinoid disease. *Acta Medica Scandinavica* **161 (supplement 334):** 7–132.

Vinik A & Moattari AR (1989) Use of somatostatin analog in management of carcinoid syndrome. *Digestive Disease Sciences* **34 (supplement):** 149–275.

Vinik A, Shih-tzer T, Moattari AR & Cheung P (1988) Somatostatin analogue (SMS 201-995) in patients with gastrinomas. *Surgery* **104:** 834–842.

von der Ohe MR, Camilleri M & Kvols LK (1994) A 5HT₃ antagonist corrects the postprandial colonic hypertonic response in carcinoid diarrhea. *Gastroenterology* **106:** 1184–1189.

von Schrenck T, Howard JM, Doppmann JL et al (1988) Prospective study of chemotherapy in patients with metastatic gastrinoma. *Gastroenterology* **94:** 1326–1334.

Wiedenmann B, Räth U, Rädsch R et al (1988) Tumour regression of an ileal carcinoid under the treatment with the somatostatin analogue SMS 201-995. *Klinische Wochenschrift* **66:** 75–77.

Wood SM, Kraenzlin MW, Adrian TE & Bloom SM (1985) Treatment of patients with pancreatic endocrine tumours using a new long-acting somatostatin analogue: symptomatic and peptide responses. *Gut* **25:** 438–444.

Yamada Y, Reisine T, Law SF et al (1992) Somatostatin receptors, an expanding family: cloning and functional characterization of human SSTRs, a protein coupled to adenyl cyclase. *Molecular Endocrinology* **6:** 2136–2142.

Yamada Y, Kagimoto S, Kubota A et al (1993) Cloning, functional expression and pharmacological characterization of a fourth (h SSTR4) and a fifth (h SSTR5) human somatostatin receptor subtype. *Biochemical and Biophysical Research Communications* **195:** 844–852.

Index

Note: Page numbers of article titles are in **bold** type.